Iron in Clinical Practice

Iron in Clinical Practice

Edited by

Sue Pavord
Oxford University Hospitals NHS Foundation Trust, Oxford, UK

Noemi Roy
Oxford University Hospitals NHS Foundation Trust, Oxford, UK

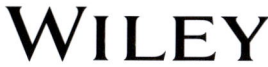

Registered Offices
John Wiley & Sons, Inc., 111 River Street, Hoboken, NJ 07030, USA
John Wiley & Sons Ltd, New Era House, 8 Oldlands Way, Bognor Regis, West Sussex, PO22 9NQ, UK

For details of our global editorial offices, customer services, and more information about Wiley products visit us at www.wiley.com.

The manufacturer's authorized representative according to the EU General Product Safety Regulation is Wiley-VCH GmbH, Boschstr. 12, 69469 Weinheim, Germany, e-mail: Product_Safety@wiley.com.

Library of Congress Cataloging-in-Publication Data applied for

Hardback ISBN: 9781394210886

Cover Design: Wiley
Cover Image: © luchschenF/Adobe Stock

Set in 9.5/12.5pt STIXTwoText by Straive, Pondicherry, India

Printed in Singapore
M126067_010425

Contents

List of Contributors   *xiii*
Preface   *xvii*
About the Companion Website   *xix*

Part 1   Introduction to Iron   *1*

1   An Introduction to Iron in the Body   *3*
Sue Pavord and Noemi Roy
Introduction   *3*
Iron in the Body   *3*
Essential Functions of Iron in the Body   *6*
Iron Deficiency   *6*
Iron Overload   *6*
Bibliography   *9*

2   Regulation of Iron Trafficking in the Body   *11*
Megan Teh and Hal Drakesmith
Introduction   *11*
Hepcidin and Systemic Iron Homeostasis   *11*
Regulation of Hepcidin   *12*
   Sensing Iron Concentrations   *12*
   Erythropoietic Demand   *14*
   Inflammation   *14*
Cellular Iron Homeostasis: Ferritin and Transferrin Receptor   *14*
Assessing Iron Status – How the Markers Used Relate to
Underlying Biology   *15*
Bibliography   *16*

3 Iron and Immunity *17*
Fabiana Busti and Domenico Girelli
Introduction *17*
The Battle for Iron and the Concept of 'Nutritional Immunity' *17*
Therapeutic Interventions Harnessing Nutritional Immunity *18*
Iron Status and Susceptibility to Infections *19*
Iron Deficiency and Health of Populations *19*
Iron Overload and Risk of Infection *20*
Iron Status and Response to Vaccines *20*
Bibliography *22*

Part 2 Iron Deficiency *23*
Part 2a Assessment and Management of Iron Deficiency *25*

4 Impact of Iron Deficiency on the Individual *27*
Patrick Kyei-Mensah
Introduction *27*
Symptoms and Signs of Iron Deficiency *28*
Impact of Iron Deficiency on Specific At-risk Groups *28*
Pregnancy, Parturition and Lactation *30*
Paediatric Population *30*
Non-pregnant Premenopausal Women *31*
Individuals from Resource-poor Settings *31*
Other Clinical Situations Associated with Iron Deficiency *31*
Gastrointestinal Bleeding *31*
Heart Failure *31*
Chronic Obstructive Airway Disease *32*
Renal Disease *32*
Conclusion *32*
Bibliography *32*

5 Assessment of Iron Deficiency *33*
Hanke L. Matlung and Dorine W. Swinkels
Introduction *33*
Definitions *33*
Ferritin Thresholds *33*
Inflammation and Liver Disease *36*
Additional Biomarkers *36*
Red Cell Indices *36*
Hepcidin Levels *37*
Conclusion *38*
Bibliography *38*

6 Available Treatments for Iron Deficiency *39*
Paolo Polzella
Introduction *39*
Oral Iron Supplementation *39*
Administration of Oral Iron *39*
Intravenous Iron Therapy *40*
Potential Adverse Effects of Intravenous Iron *41*
Individualising Treatment *42*
Bibliography *43*

Part 2b Causes, Impact, Management and Prevention of Iron Deficiency in Clinical Specialties *45*

7 Iron Deficiency in Primary Care *47*
David McCartney
Introduction *47*
Presentation of Iron Deficiency in Primary Care *47*
The Main Causes of Iron Deficiency in Primary Care *48*
Pre-menopausal Women *48*
Post-menopausal Women and Men *49*
Older Adults *49*
The Diagnosis of Iron Deficiency in Primary Care *49*
Haemoglobin *49*
Iron Studies *49*
Further Investigations *50*
Treatment of Iron Deficiency in Primary Care *50*
Dietary Advice and Prevention of Future Iron Deficiency *51*
Bibliography *51*

8 Iron Deficiency in the Preoperative Patient *53*
Caroline R. Evans
Introduction *53*
Haemoglobin Thresholds *53*
Causes of Iron Deficiency in the Surgical Setting *54*
Laboratory Tests *54*
Management of Preoperative Iron Deficiency *55*
Iron Treatment *55*
Postoperative Management *56*
Conclusion *56*
Bibliography *56*

9 Iron Deficiency in Gastroenterology *57*
Mohmmed Tauseef Sharip and Nurulamin M. Noor
Introduction *57*
Gastrointestinal Causes of Iron Deficiency *57*
Assessment of Iron Deficiency in Patients with Gastrointestinal Disease *59*
Specific Gastrointestinal Investigations *59*
Angiodysplasia *62*
Treatment of Iron Deficiency in Patients with Gastrointestinal Disease *62*
Bibliography *64*

10 Iron Deficiency in Renal Medicine *65*
Philip A. Kalra
Introduction *65*
Types of Iron Used in Nephrology and Safety Considerations *65*
Iron Use in Haemodialysis Patients *66*
Iron Use in Non-Dialysis-Dependent Chronic Kidney Disease *68*
Iron Use in Peritoneal Dialysis *68*
Bibliography *69*

11 Iron Deficiency in Cardiology *71*
Samira Lakhal-Littleton
Introduction *71*
Causes of Iron Deficiency in Heart Failure *71*
Impact of Iron Deficiency in Heart Failure *72*
Management of Iron Deficiency in Heart Failure *72*
Diagnostic and Management Uncertainties in Individuals with Cardiac Disease *73*
  Current Definitions of Iron Deficiency *73*
Current Iron Replacement Therapies *74*
Bibliography *75*

12 Iron Deficiency in Neurology *77*
Carmen Jacob and Ian Galea
Introduction *77*
Iron Utilisation in the Central Nervous System *77*
Iron and Neurocognitive Development *79*
Neurological Associations in Iron Deficiency *79*
Recommendations for Management of Iron Deficiency with Neurological
Symptoms *80*
Conclusion *80*
Bibliography *80*

13 Iron Deficiency in Obstetrics *83*
Sue Pavord
Introduction *83*
The Maternal Effects of Iron Deficiency *83*

Fetal Effects of Iron Deficiency   *85*
Defining Anaemia in Pregnancy   *85*
How Is Iron Deficiency Diagnosed in Pregnancy?   *86*
Indications for Intravenous Iron   *86*
Management of Postpartum Anaemia   *87*
Bibliography   *87*

14   Iron Deficiency in Gynaecology   *89*
Imo J. Akpan
Introduction   *89*
Causes of Heavy Menstrual Bleeding   *89*
Definition of Heavy Menstrual Bleeding   *89*
Prevention of Iron Deficiency in Gynaecology   *89*
Investigation of Heavy Menstrual Bleeding   *90*
Management of Heavy Menstrual Bleeding   *91*
   Hormonal Preparations   *91*
   Anticoagulation Modification   *91*
   Haemostatic Agents   *92*
   Surgical Management   *92*
Iron Deficiency and Iron Deficiency Anaemia in Gynaecology   *92*
Impact of Iron Deficiency in Gynaecology   *92*
Management of Iron Deficiency in Women with Gynaecological Bleeding   *94*
   Oral Iron Supplementation   *94*
   Parenteral Iron Supplementation   *95*
   Blood Transfusion   *95*
Bibliography   *95*

15   Iron Deficiency in Orthopaedics   *97*
Antony Palmer
Introduction   *97*
Diagnosis   *97*
Aetiology of Iron Deficiency   *98*
Preoperative Treatment of Iron Deficiency Anaemia   *98*
Patient Outcomes   *98*
Iron Deficiency Without Anaemia   *100*
Bibliography   *100*

16   Iron Deficiency in Intensive Care   *101*
Akshay Shah
Introduction   *101*
Iron Homeostasis in Critical Illness   *101*
Diagnosing Iron Deficiency in Critical Illness   *103*
Clinical Implications of Iron Deficiency in Intensive Care Unit   *103*
Patient Blood Management in Intensive Care   *104*
Intravenous Iron in Intensive Care   *104*

Concomitant Therapies for Anaemia Management in Intensive Care *104*
Bibliography *105*

17 Iron Deficiency in Medical Oncology *107*
Sue Pavord
Introduction *107*
Causes of Anaemia in Patients with Cancer *107*
Diagnosis of Iron Deficiency in Patients with Cancer *108*
Management of Anaemia in Patients with Cancer *108*
Erythropoiesis Stimulating Agents *108*
Blood Transfusion in Oncology *109*
Prevention of Anaemia in Patients with Cancer *109*
Implementation of Local Policy *109*
Novel Anti-anaemia Agents *110*
Conclusion *110*
Bibliography *111*

Part 3 Iron Overload *113*
Part 3a Causes of Iron Overload *115*

18 Transfusional Iron Overload *117*
Samah Babiker and John Porter
Introduction *117*
The Causes of Iron Overload and Influencing Factors *117*
Pathophysiology and Effects of Transfusional Iron Loading on Body Iron
Distribution *117*
Rates of Transfusional Iron Overloading and Distribution in Different Diseases *119*
Consequences of Transfusional Iron Overload *119*
Prevention of Transfusional Iron Overload *121*
Bibliography *121*

19 Haemochromatosis *123*
Graca Porto
Introduction *123*
Pathogenesis *123*
Frequency and Penetrance of *HFE*-Related Haemochromatosis *124*
Diagnosis *125*
Treatment and Prevention *127*
Bibliography *127*

20 Ineffective Erythropoiesis *129*
Noémi Roy
Introduction *129*
Erythropoiesis *129*

The Role of Erythropoietin and Iron   *130*
Ferrokinetic Studies   *131*
Erythroferrone   *131*
Bibliography   *132*

Part 3b   Effects of Iron Overload on Body Organs   *133*

21   Iron Overload in the Heart   *135*
Malcolm Walker
Iron and the Heart   *135*
Cardiac Iron Regulation   *135*
Iron Overload   *135*
Clinical Presentations and Their Management   *136*
   Ventricular Dysfunction and Heart Failure   *136*
   Arrhythmia   *137*
Assessment of Cardiac Iron   *137*
   Magnetic Resonance Imaging   *137*
   Other Heart Tests   *138*
Long-Term Management and Prevention   *138*
Bibliography   *140*

22   Iron Overload and the Liver   *141*
Emma Saunsbury and Jeremy Cobbold
Introduction   *141*
Histological Patterns of Hepatic Iron Overload   *141*
Pathophysiology of Hepatic Damage Secondary to Iron Overload   *141*
Assessment of Hepatic Iron Overload   *143*
Bibliography   *144*

23   Impact of Iron Overload on the Endocrine System   *147*
Amy Morrison and Miles Levy
Introduction   *147*
Diabetes Mellitus   *147*
Reproductive Endocrinology   *148*
Growth and Bone Health   *150*
Adrenal Function   *150*
Summary   *151*
Bibliography   *152*

24   Iron Overload and the Musculoskeletal System   *153*
Kassim Javaid
Introduction   *153*
Osteoporosis and Fracture Risk   *153*
Osteoarthritis   *154*

Calcium Pyrophosphate Deposition Disease   *155*
Management of Iron Overload in the Joints   *155*
Bibliography   *156*

Part 3c   Assessment and Management of Iron Overload   *157*

25   Assessment of Iron Overload   *159*
Subarna Chakravorty
Introduction   *159*
Awareness of Potential Causes   *159*
Assessment of Transfusional Iron Overload   *159*
Role of Serum Ferritin and Iron Studies in Assessing Iron Overload   *160*
Imaging in Iron Overload   *161*
Monitoring Requirements for At-risk Patients   *162*
Bibliography   *163*

26   Management of Iron Overload   *165*
Nandini Sadasivam
Introduction   *165*
Iron Chelation Therapy   *165*
Indications for Iron Chelation Therapy   *165*
Administration of Iron Chelation Therapy   *166*
Combination Chelation Therapy   *166*
  When to Start Iron Chelation Therapy   *168*
  Practical Tips for Clinicians   *168*
    Desferrioxamine   *168*
    Deferasirox   *169*
    Deferiprone   *169*
Calculation of ROIL Adults   *169*
Calculation of ROIL in Paediatric   *169*
Practical Prescribing Tips   *170*
Dose Adjustments for Comorbidities   *171*
  Renal Disease   *171*
    Desferrioxamine   *171*
    Deferasirox   *171*
    Established Dialysis   *171*
  Liver Disease   *171*
    Deferasirox   *171*
  Pregnancy   *171*
Emerging Novel Therapies   *171*
Bibliography   *172*

Index   *173*

List of Contributors

Imo J. Akpan
Department of Medicine, Division of
Haematology/Oncology, Columbia
University Irving Medical Center
New York, NY, USA

Samah Babiker
Evelina London Children's Hospital
St Thomas' Hospital
London, UK

Fabiana Busti
Department of Medicine, Section
of Internal Medicine, University of
Verona Italy

Veneto Region Referral Center for Iron
Disorders and European Reference
Network Center for Rare Hematological
Diseases "EuroBloodNet"

Subarna Chakravorty
Department of Paediatric Haematology
King's College Hospital
London, UK

Jeremy Cobbold
Department of Gastroenterology and
Hepatology
Oxford University Hospitals NHS
Foundation Trust, Oxford, UK

Hal Drakesmith
Medical Research Council Translational
Immune Discovery Unit, MRC Weatherall
Institute of Molecular Medicine, University
of Oxford, John Radcliffe Hospital
Headington, Oxford, UK

Caroline R. Evans
Department of Anaesthetics, Cardiff
and Vale University Healthboard
Cardiff, UK

Ian Galea
Clinical Neurosciences, Clinical and
Experimental Sciences, Faculty of
Medicine, University of Southampton, UK

Wessex Neurological Centre, University
Hospital Southampton NHS Foundation
Trust, UK

Domenico Girelli
Department of Medicine, Section
of Internal Medicine, University of
Verona Italy

Veneto Region Referral Center for Iron
Disorders and European Reference
Network Center for Rare Hematological
Diseases "EuroBloodNet"

Carmen Jacob
Clinical Neurosciences, Clinical and
Experimental Sciences, Faculty of
Medicine, University of Southampton, UK

Wessex Neurological Centre, University
Hospital Southampton NHS Foundation
Trust, UK

Kassim Javaid
The Botnar Centre, Nuffield Orthopaedic
Centre, Oxford, UK

Philip A. Kalra
Department of Nephrology, Salford Royal
Hospital, Northern Care Alliance NHS
Foundation Trust, UK

Patrick Kyei-Mensah
Department of Haematology, Oxford
University Hospitals NHS Foundation
Trust, Oxford, UK

Samira Lakhal-Littleton
Department of Physiology, Anatomy and
Genetics, University of Oxford
Oxford, UK

Miles Levy
Department of Diabetes & Endocrinology
University Hospitals of Leicester NHS
Trust,
Leicester, UK

Hanke L. Matlung
Sanquin Research and
Landsteiner Laboratory
Department of Molecular Hematology
Amsterdam, the Netherlands

David McCartney
School of Medicine and Biomedical
Sciences, Medical Sciences Division
University of Oxford Academic Centre
John Radcliffe Hospital
Oxford, UK

Amy Morrison
Department of Diabetes & Endocrinology
University Hospitals of Leicester NHS
Trust
Leicester, UK

Nurulamin M. Noor
Department of Gastroenterology
Cambridge University Hospitals NHS
Foundation Trust, Cambridge, UK

Department of Medicine, University of
Cambridge School of Clinical Medicine
Cambridge, UK

Antony Palmer
Department of Surgery, Nuffield Orthopaedic
Hospital, Oxford University Hospitals NHS
Foundation Trust, Oxford, UK

Sue Pavord
Department of Haematology, Oxford
University Hospitals NHS Foundation
Trust, Oxford, UK

Paolo Polzella
Department of Haematology, Oxford
University Hospitals NHS Foundation Trust
Oxford, UK

John Porter
Department of Haematology
University College Hospital
London, UK

Graca Porto
Hematology Serviço de Imuno-
hemoterapia, CHUdSA-Centro Hospitalar
Universitário de Santo António
Porto, Portugal

Noemi Roy
Department of Haematology, Oxford
University Hospitals NHS Foundation
Trust, Oxford, UK

Nandini Sadasivam
Department of Haematology
Manchester Royal Infirmary
Manchester, UK

Emma Saunsbury
Department of Gastroenterology and
Hepatology
Oxford University Hospitals NHS
Foundation Trust
Oxford, UK

Akshay Shah
Nuffield Department of Clinical
Neurosciences, University of Oxford
Oxford University Hospitals NHS
Foundation Trust
Oxford, UK

Department of Anaesthesia
Hammersmith Hospital
Imperial College Healthcare NHS Trust
London, UK

Mohmmed Tauseef Sharip
Department of Gastroenterology
Cambridge University Hospitals NHS
Foundation Trust, Cambridge, UK

Dorine W. Swinkels
Sanquin Blood Bank
Amsterdam, the Netherlands

Department of Laboratory Medicine
Radboud University Medical Center
Nijmegen, the Netherlands

Megan Teh
Medical Research Council Translational
Immune Discovery Unit, MRC Weatherall
Institute of Molecular Medicine, University
of Oxford, John Radcliffe Hospital
Headington, Oxford, UK

Malcolm Walker
Hatter Cardiovascular Institute, University
College London Hospital
London, UK

Preface

Sue Pavord and Noemi Roy

Department of Haematology, Oxford University Hospitals NHS Foundation Trust, Oxford, UK

"It is the greatest happiness of the greatest number that is the measure of right and wrong."

The utilitarian approach of Jeremy Bentham, who stated this in reference to morals and legislation, can be applied to medical practice.

Iron disorders are common. Effective management of them ensures fitness and resilience throughout an individual's life cycle – the fetal and neonatal period, growth and development, educational years, work productivity, pregnancy, aging, medical disease, and surgery.

The provision of healthcare is increasingly challenged by the advancing age and progressive diversity of populations. Maintaining optimal health for as long as possible is crucial for individuals and their families.

Recognition and management of iron disorders is one of the best examples of preventative medicine and paramount for population health.

We developed this book to raise awareness of iron disorders which are highly prevalent, disabling, underdiagnosed, and undertreated.

The book aims to provide healthcare professionals with a comprehensive guide to the role of iron in the body, recognising and diagnosing iron disorders and implementing successful treatment strategies.

This book should serve as a valuable resource for improving knowledge and skills in managing iron deficiency and iron overload.

The book is based on the latest available evidence. There remain gaps in our knowledge, which will continue to be filled over the coming years.

We thank all the contributors who have given up their time to generously share their specific knowledge and expertise.

About the Companion Website

This book is accompanied by a companion website:

www.wiley.com/go/medicine5e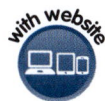

The website includes:

- MCQs

Part 1

Introduction to Iron

1

An Introduction to Iron in the Body

Sue Pavord and Noemi Roy

Department of Haematology, Oxford University Hospitals NHS Foundation Trust, Oxford, UK

Introduction

Iron is the most common element on Earth. In the Earth's crust it is the fourth most abundant element after oxygen, silicon and aluminium, being mainly deposited by meteorites in its metallic state. As life evolved, organisms selected from available elements for fundamental physiological processes, and iron has been utilised by every living organism and is essential for a multitude of biological functions.

Humans have evolved structures to bind iron as well as using free iron ions (Figure 1.1). Iron participates in vital metabolic processes of every body cell, including oxygen transport, catalytic enzyme activity, electron transport, deoxyribonucleic acid (DNA) synthesis and cell proliferation. Cellular iron is predominantly located in the mitochondria and endoplasmic reticulum. In humans, 2% of genes encode an iron protein, and these genes are more frequently associated with pathologies than all other human genes.

Iron in the Body

An average sized human body will contain about 4g iron, an approximate concentration of 50mg/kg. Table 1.1 shows a rough distribution of iron in the body.

The daily intake of iron from a balanced diet is around 2mg. This equals the daily losses from sweat and shedding of epithelial cells such as skin and intestinal cells so that iron is maintained in a physiological range. Iron is conserved in the body by recycling, a function of the reticuloendothelial system.

When released into the plasma from intestinal cells (following absorption from the gut) and reticuloendothelial macrophages (from phagocytosis of senescent red cells), it is captured by transferrin and delivered to the tissues. The iron-bound transferrin attaches to the

Iron in Clinical Practice, First Edition. Edited by Sue Pavord and Noemi Roy.
© 2025 John Wiley & Sons Ltd. Published 2025 by John Wiley & Sons Ltd.
Companion website: www.wiley.com/go/medicine5e

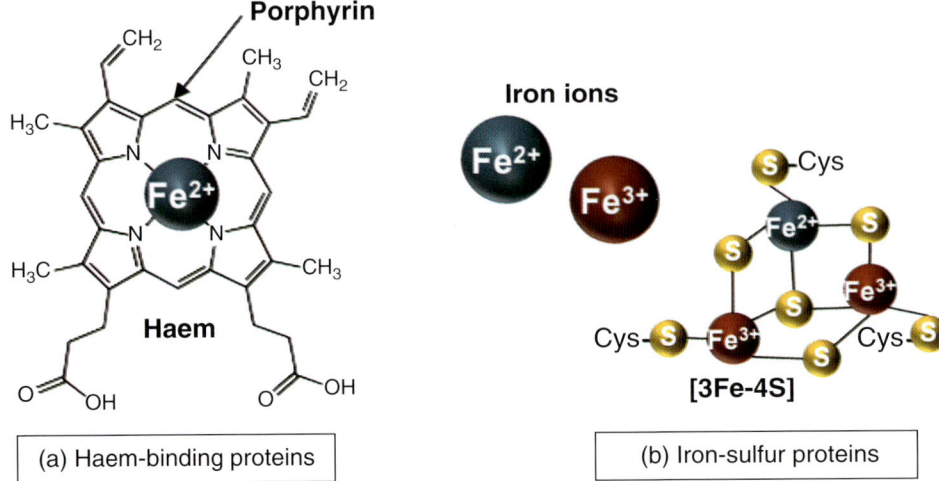

(a) Haem-binding proteins

(b) Iron-sulfur proteins

Figure 1.1 Iron-containing proteins.

Table 1.1 Distribution of iron in the body.

	Percentage of total body iron
Oxygen transport and storage	
Haemoglobin	60–70%
Myoglobin	10%
Energy generation	
Mitochondrial cytochromes of electron transport chain; elements of citric acid cycle	~1%
Key enzymatic processes	
Cytochrome P450 and other metabolic pathways	
Synthesis	
Catecholamine, neurotransmitter, melanin and collagen synthesis	
Immune cell function	
Storage	
Ferritin, haemosiderin	20–30%
Transport	
Transferrin	<0.2%

transferrin receptor (TfR) on the surface of cells, and its iron is internalised into the cell. Once inside the cell, iron is transported to mitochondria for the synthesis of haem or iron–sulphur clusters, which are integral parts of several metalloproteins. Surplus iron is stored and detoxified in ferritin (Figure 1.2).

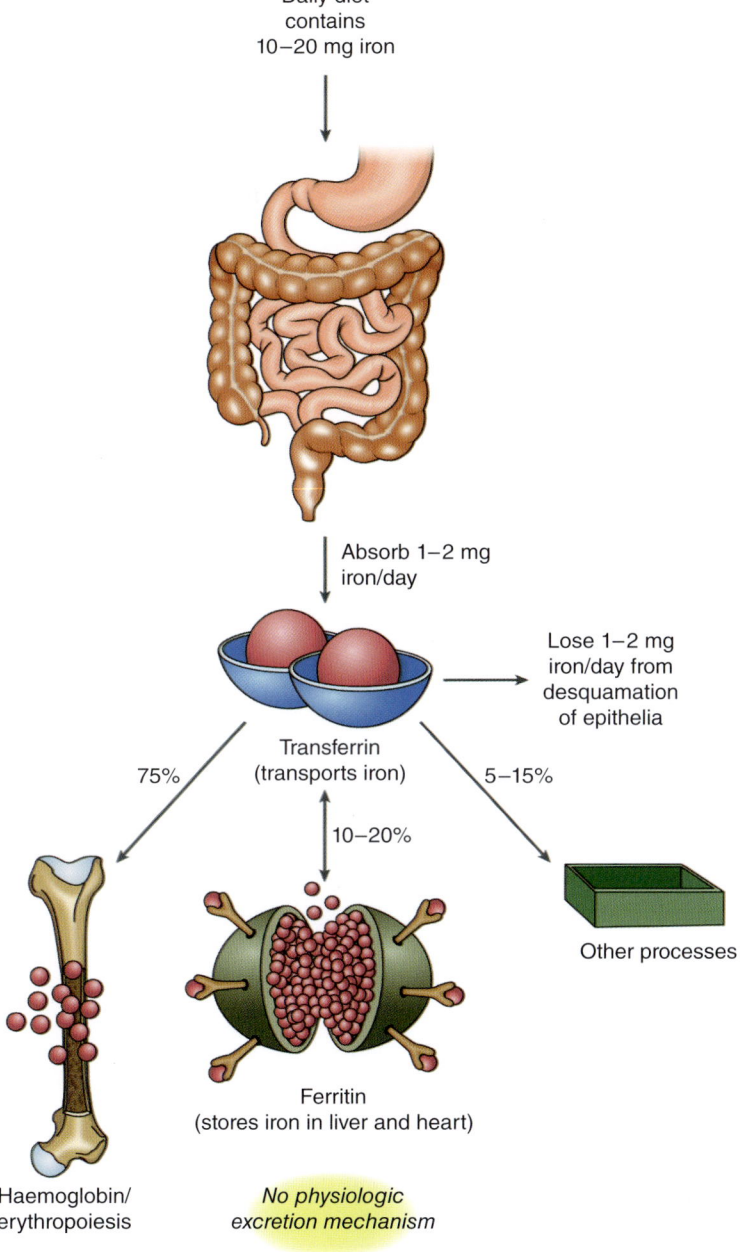

Figure 1.2 Iron utilisation.

Essential Functions of Iron in the Body

Approximately 70% of the iron is used by the bone marrow to make haemoglobin (Hb). This is synthesised by erythroblasts, which show high expression of TfRs. The erythroblast matures into a reticulocyte and ultimately to an erythrocyte (Figure 1.3). Around 8% of the iron is used in myoglobin, another haemoprotein responsible for oxygen binding and transport but specific to cardiac and skeletal muscle.

Iron is also required as a cofactor for many non-haem proteins, including catalase and peroxidase enzymes, which take part in oxygen metabolism, and cytochromes, which are involved in electron transport and mitochondrial respiration. These non-haem iron-containing proteins have crucial functions, as they are used in DNA synthesis, gene regulation, cell proliferation and differentiation, hormone synthesis and drug metabolism. In the brain and nervous system, iron is required for neurotransmitter synthesis, myelin synthesis and development and metabolism of brain cells (Figure 1.4). The blood–brain barrier modulates iron levels in the brain.

Genetic and acquired diseases of the tissues and organs involved in iron utilisation and recycling cause a dysregulation of the iron cycle and may lead to iron deficiency or excess. Both have a negative impact on health.

Iron Deficiency

Iron deficiency (ID) is a global health concern, affecting more than four billion people worldwide. It is the most common nutritional deficiency in low- and middle-income countries and in high-income countries.

According to World Health Organisation (WHO) statistics, ID anaemia affects 30% of the world population, 40% of all children aged 6–59 months, 37% of pregnant women and 30% of all women aged 15–49 years. Because of its very wide prevalence, ID imposes a considerable burden of morbidity on a significant proportion of the world population.

In 2019, the WHO estimated the loss of about 50 million healthy life years, as a consequence of disability from ID. An earlier statistic from the WHO Global Burden of Disease Project 2000 (GBD 2000) estimated over 840,000 deaths worldwide as a direct consequence of ID, with the majority seen in parts of Asia and Africa.

Iron Overload

Iron is highly conserved in the body; there is no mechanism for excretion. Apart from the small amount of iron lost from sweat and desquamation, it is only through bleeding that iron is lost. Thus, there are many disease states where iron accumulates. These include inherited or acquired abnormalities of erythropoiesis, where iron uptake into the erythroblast is ineffective, exacerbated by the need for frequent transfusion. Each unit of blood transfused contains around 250 mg iron.

Deposition of excess iron in body tissues can cause significant harm. Iron is a transitional metal and in changing its charge between ferrous (Fe^{2+}) and ferric (Fe^{3+}) forms, unstable

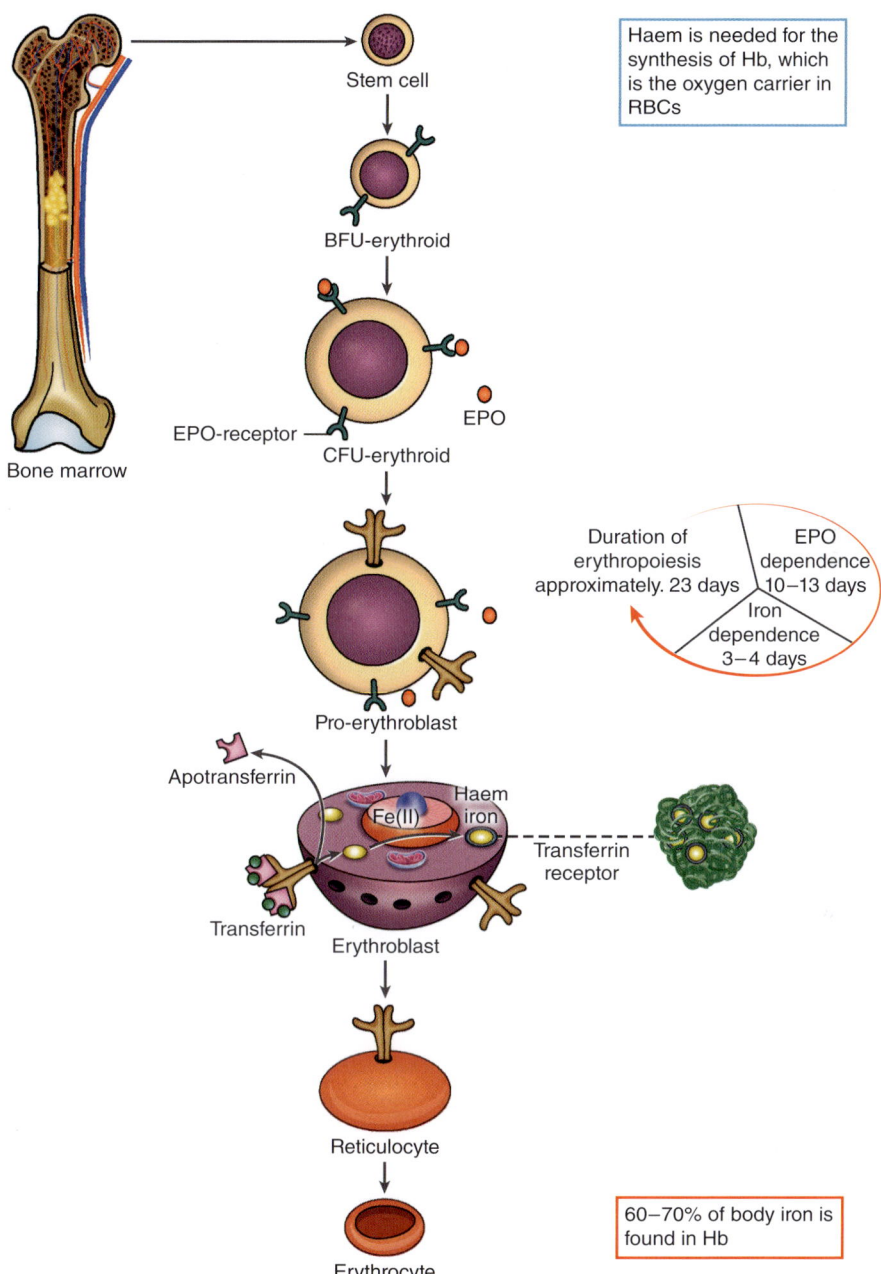

Haem is needed for the synthesis of Hb, which is the oxygen carrier in RBCs

Stem cell

BFU-erythroid

EPO-receptor

EPO

CFU-erythroid

Bone marrow

Duration of erythropoiesis approximately. 23 days

EPO dependence 10–13 days

Iron dependence 3–4 days

Pro-erythroblast

Apotransferrin

Fe(II)

Haem iron

Transferrin receptor

Transferrin

Erythroblast

Reticulocyte

60–70% of body iron is found in Hb

Erythrocyte

Figure 1.3 Stages of red cell maturation where iron is utilised for haem synthesis. BFU, burst-forming unit; CFU, colony-forming unit; EPO, erythropoietin; Hb, haemoglobin; RBC, red blood cell. *Source:* Figure adapted from Besarab et al. (2009) and Geissler and Singh (2011).

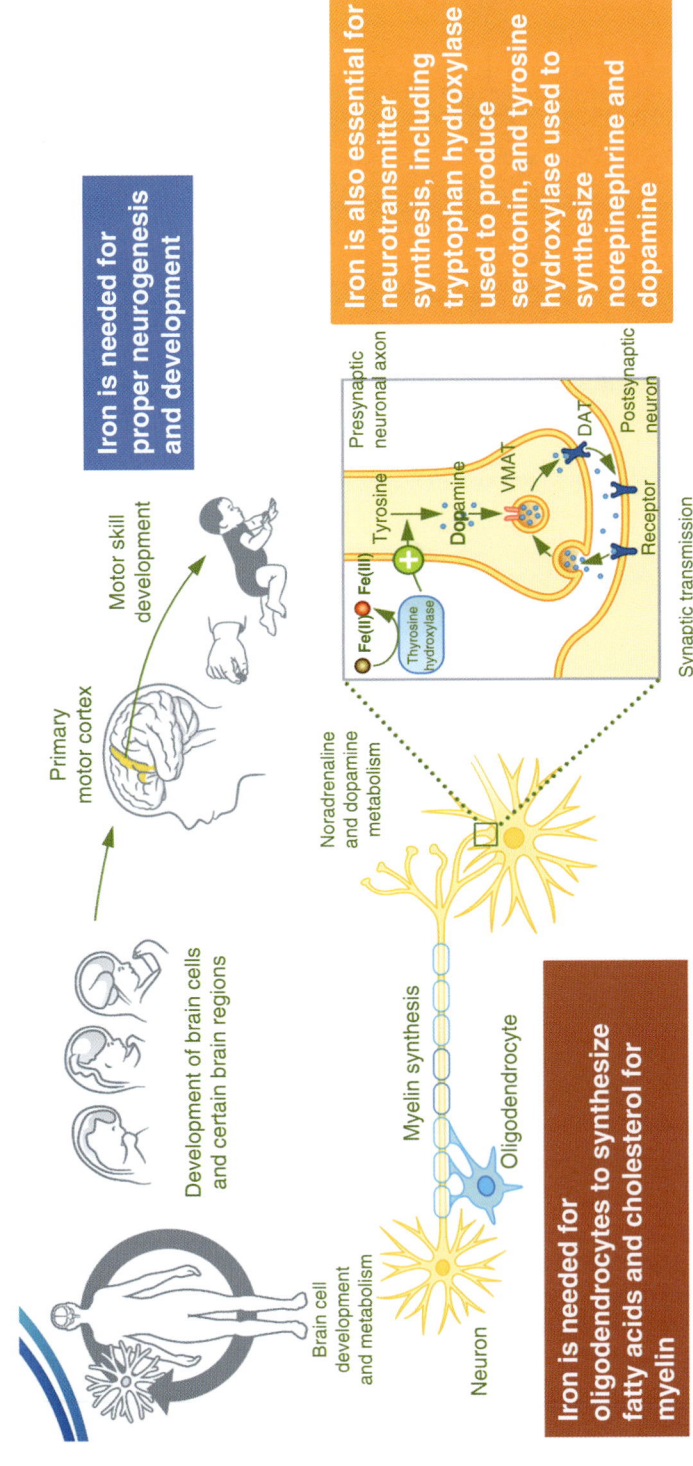

Iron is needed for proper neurogenesis and development

Iron is also essential for neurotransmitter synthesis, including tryptophan hydroxylase used to produce serotonin, and tyrosine hydroxylase used to synthesize norepinephrine and dopamine

Iron is needed for oligodendrocytes to synthesize fatty acids and cholesterol for myelin

Primary motor cortex

Motor skill development

Development of brain cells and certain brain regions

Brain cell development and metabolism

Myelin synthesis

Noradrenaline and dopamine metabolism

Neuron

Oligodendrocyte

Presynaptic neuronal axon

Tyrosine

Dopamine

VMAT

DAT

Postsynaptic neuron

Receptor

Fe(II) Fe(III)

Thyrosine hydroxylase

Synaptic transmission

Figure 1.4 Iron requirements in the nervous system. DAT, dopamine transporter; VMAT, vesicular monoamine transporter. *Source:* Figure adapted from Radlowski and Johnson (2013).

Figure 1.5 Release of unpaired electrons (free radicals) during transition between its divalent ferrous form (Fe^{2+}) and its trivalent ferric (Fe^{3+}) form.

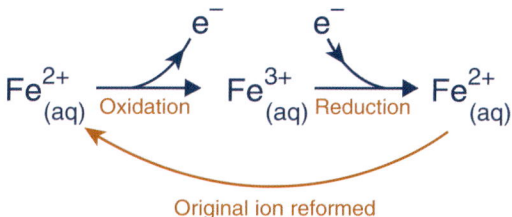

$$Fe^{2+}_{(aq)} \xrightarrow{\quad\text{Oxidation}\quad} Fe^{3+}_{(aq)} \xrightarrow{\quad\text{Reduction}\quad} Fe^{2+}_{(aq)}$$

Original ion reformed

and highly reactive free radicals are released, which can be toxic to tissues (Figure 1.5). They can react with other molecules in cells causing damage to DNA, RNA, lipids and proteins and may lead to cell death.

In summary, whilst regulatory mechanisms are in place to maintain physiological iron levels, these can easily be overcome by even minor disturbance, and both ID and iron excess are commonly encountered in clinical practice.

The chapters in this book will review the functions of iron, iron homeostasis, inflammation and the acute phase response, the causes and clinical impact of iron disorders, determination of iron status and treatment options for ID and iron overload.

Bibliography

Abbaspour, N., Hurrell, R., and Kelishadi, R. (2014). Review on iron and its importance for human health. *J Res Med Sci* 19: 164–174.

Andreini, C., Putignano, V., Rosato, A., and Banci, L. (2018). The human iron-proteome. *Metallomics* 10: 1223–1231.

Besarab, A., Hörl, W.H., and Silverberg, D. (2009). Iron metabolism, iron deficiency, thrombocytosis, and the cardiorenal anemia syndrome. *Oncologist* 14 (Suppl 1): 22.

Geissler, C. and Singh, M. (2011). Iron, meat and health. *Nutrients* 3: 283–316.

Kulaszyńska, M., Kwiatkowski, S., and Skonieczna-Żydecka, K. (2024). The iron metabolism with a specific focus on the functioning of the nervous system. *Biomedicines* 12: 595.

Lieu, P.T., Heiskala, M., Peterson, P.A., and Yang, Y. (2001). The roles of iron in health and disease. *Mol Aspects Med* 22: 1–87.

Radlowski, E.C. and Johnson, R.W. (2013). Perinatal iron deficiency and neurocognitive development. *Front Hum Neurosci* 7: 585.

Yiannikourides, A. and Latunde-Dada, G.O. (2019). A short review of iron metabolism and pathophysiology of iron disorders. *Medicines* 6: 85.

2

Regulation of Iron Trafficking in the Body

Megan Teh and Hal Drakesmith

Medical Research Council Translational Immune Discovery Unit, MRC Weatherall Institute of Molecular Medicine, University of Oxford, John Radcliffe Hospital, Headington, Oxford, UK

Introduction

Iron carries oxygen in haemoglobin, facilitates energy generation by oxidative phosphorylation and catalyses redox reactions by many different enzymes. As a result, iron is a critical co-factor for life, whilst iron deficiency has multiple complex effects. Moreover, because of its reactive nature, excess iron generates harmful reactive species such as the hydroxyl radical that damages proteins, lipids and DNA. Therefore, maintaining iron homeostasis is vital and occurs at systemic and cellular levels. Notably, iron excretion is not regulated, instead body iron is controlled by absorption from the diet and recycling of iron from aged red blood cells.

Hepcidin and Systemic Iron Homeostasis

Hepcidin is a 25 amino acid peptide hormone secreted primarily from the liver into the circulation. The 'receptor' for hepcidin is a multi-transmembrane protein called ferroportin, which mediates iron efflux from cells. Hepcidin directly and specifically binds ferroportin, inhibits its action and causes its degradation. Therefore, hepcidin prevents iron export from cells. See Figure 2.1.

The cells that have most ferroportin are the duodenal enterocytes and red pulp macrophages in the spleen. Many other cell types including hepatocytes, cardiomyocytes, syncytiotrophoblasts and immune cells also express ferroportin. By inhibiting ferroportin activity, hepcidin impairs uptake of iron from food and recycling of iron from senescent erythrocytes, inhibits release of stored liver iron, affects heart iron content and modulates transfer of iron across the placenta.

High hepcidin decreases the concentration of iron in plasma (transferrin saturation drops), but increases iron in the spleen, whilst low hepcidin allows ferroportin to freely export iron, increasing transferrin saturation. Thus, the amount of hepcidin that the liver

Iron in Clinical Practice, First Edition. Edited by Sue Pavord and Noemi Roy.
© 2025 John Wiley & Sons Ltd. Published 2025 by John Wiley & Sons Ltd.
Companion website: www.wiley.com/go/medicine5e

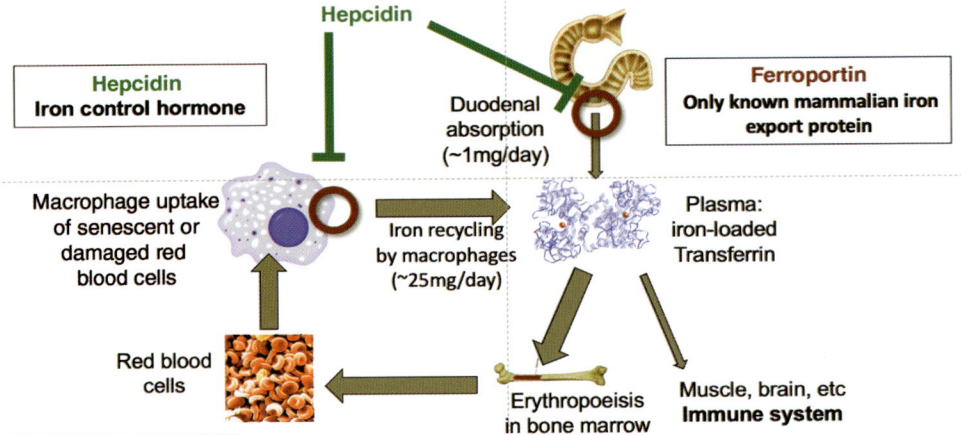

Figure 2.1 Overview of the regulation of ferroportin and iron trafficking by hepcidin. Around 1 mg of iron is absorbed from the diet daily, through duodenal enterocytes. The final step of iron transport from enterocytes into the circulation is via ferroportin, the only known cellular iron exporter. In plasma, iron atoms are tightly bound by the protein transferrin, which then delivers iron to cells that express the transferrin receptor. Although all human cell types require iron (including muscle, brain and the immune system), the major demand for iron at steady-state in adults is for erythropoiesis. Iron is incorporated into the haem of haemoglobin in red blood cells; these cells survive for around 120 days in humans, after which they are phagocytosed by macrophages (mostly in the spleen) and degraded. The iron is released from haem and recycled into the circulation via ferroportin. Around 25 mg of iron is recycled per day. The iron regulatory hormone hepcidin, secreted from the liver, binds and blocks ferroportin and induces its destruction. Therefore the concentration of circulating hepcidin controls both the amount of iron absorbed from the diet and the efficiency of iron recycling, affecting the total amount of iron in the body and its distribution.

secretes controls both the level of iron in the body and the inter-tissue compartmentalisation of iron.

Common genetic defects that impair hepcidin synthesis cause iron overload (e.g. in haemochromatosis and thalassaemia), whilst rare mutations that cause hepcidin overexpression cause severe iron deficiency that is refractory to oral iron supplements.

Regulation of Hepcidin

The control of hepcidin synthesis is vital for maintenance of overall body iron homeostasis (Figure 2.2). The physiological mechanisms that determine hepcidin production can be split into three overall inputs: sensing iron concentrations, erythropoietic demand for iron and inflammation.

Sensing Iron Concentrations

The liver senses iron availability in two ways: transferrin saturation and iron stores. Transferrin-bound iron is directly sensed by a receptor complex on hepatocytes. Transferrin iron, acting via this receptor complex, modulates binding of and signalling by soluble

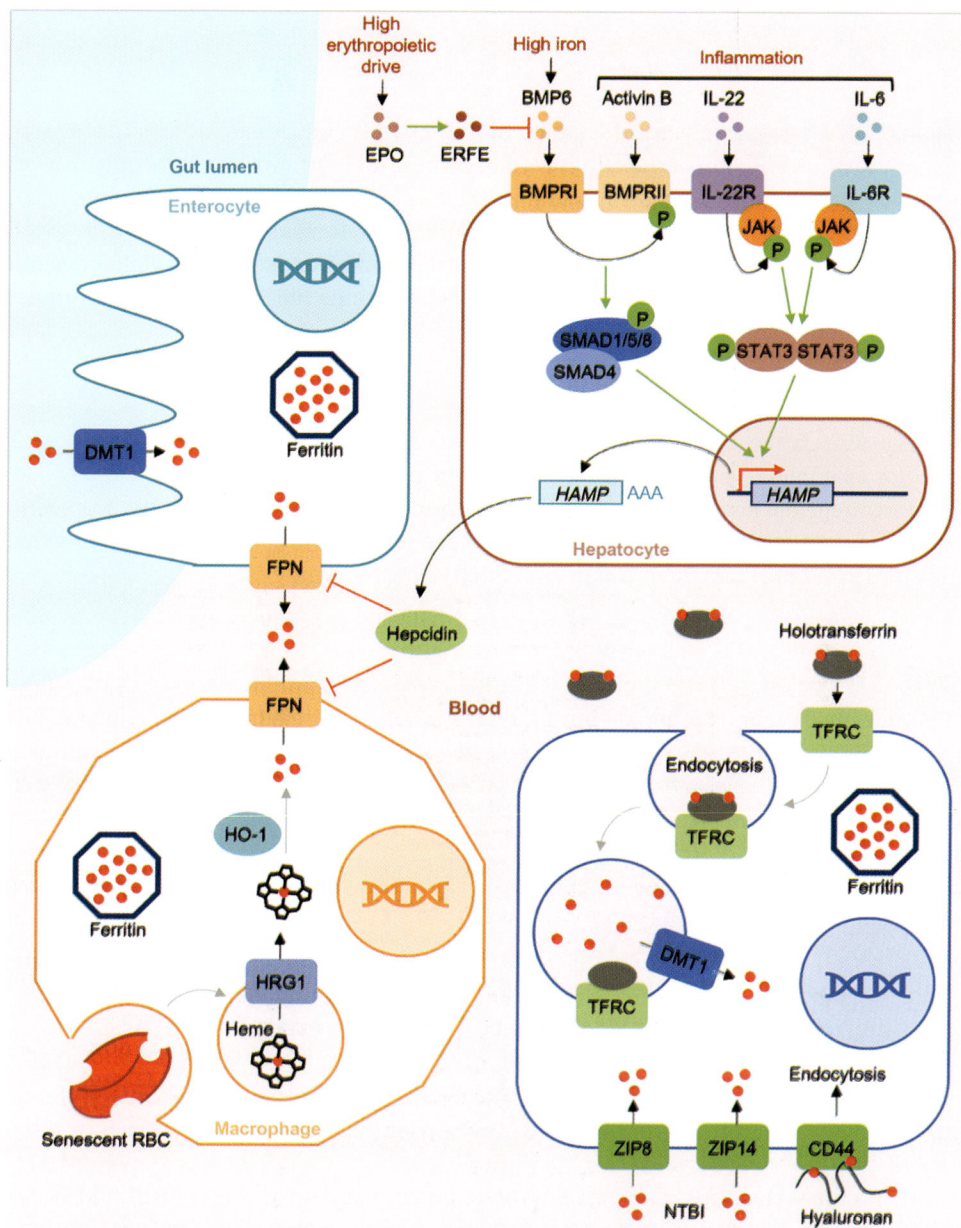

Figure 2.2 Control of hepcidin synthesis and cellular iron uptake mechanisms. Iron is taken up by enterocytes from the lumen of the gut by divalent metal transporter 1 (DMT1) and released into the circulation by ferroportin (FPN) or be stored in ferritin. Macrophages recycle the iron from phagocytosed senescent red blood cells (RBCs). RBCs are degraded and haem is released into the cytosol by haem-responsive gene-1 (HRG1). The enzyme haemoxygenase-1 (HO-1) subsequently degrades haem releasing the iron ions which enter the blood via FPN. Serum iron is controlled by hepatic hepcidin which inhibits iron release into the serum by FPN. Hepcidin is induced by high iron by bone morphogenetic protein-6 (BMP6) and by inflammation by interleukin (IL)-6, IL-22 and activin B. IL-22 and IL-6 activate a JAK-STAT3 phosphorylation cascade to induce hepcidin upregulation. High erythropoietic drive induces erythropoietin (EPO) and erythroferrone (ERFE) sequentially which suppresses hepcidin via BMP-6 inhibition. BMP signalling induces SMAD1/5/8 phosphorylation and recruitment of SMAD4 to upregulate hepcidin transcription. Transferrin receptor (TFRC) binding to iron-bound transferrin induces endocytosis for iron uptake. Endosome acidification releases the iron from transferrin and the iron can enter the cytosol via DMT1. Non-transferrin-bound iron (NTBI) can also enter the cell via Zrt-/Irt-like protein (ZIP)-8 or ZIP-14. Hyaluronan bound iron can be taken up by binding of CD44 and subsequent endocytosis.

proteins called bone morphogenetic proteins (BMPs). BMP induces an intracellular signalling pathway that enhances transcription and synthesis of hepcidin. The BMPs themselves are made by neighbouring liver sinusoidal epithelial cells in response to cellular iron accumulation. The way in which liver sinusoidal epithelial cells sense iron stores is not well understood. Overall, increasing transferrin saturation and iron stores stimulate hepcidin concentration, and hepcidin limits iron absorption, returning the system to equilibrium.

Erythropoietic Demand

Erythropoiesis is the most iron-requiring process in the body. Increased erythropoietic drive (for example, in pregnancy, after blood loss, hypoxic conditions or red cell defects) suppresses hepcidin and facilitates iron absorption and release of iron stores. Erythropoietin (EPO) stimulates developing red blood cells to secrete a protein called erythroferrone that binds BMPs and prevents them from stimulating hepcidin synthesis.

Inflammation

When infection occurs, the innate immune system releases inflammatory mediators, one of which, interleukin-6, is a potent inducer of hepcidin synthesis. Increased hepcidin then causes a profound decrease in plasma iron, which is protective against blood-borne extracellular pathogens, which require iron to proliferate. However, inflammation caused by other types of pathogens, and sterile inflammation, can also induce hepcidin by the same pathway, and in these circumstances persistently increased hepcidin contributes to the anaemia of inflammation.

Cellular Iron Homeostasis: Ferritin and Transferrin Receptor

In addition to systemic iron homeostasis, there are cell-intrinsic mechanisms that help individual cells maintain iron balance. Cells contain many different types of iron sensors.

Two important iron sensors are called iron regulatory proteins 1 and 2 (IRP1 and IRP2). Their iron regulation functions are activated by low cellular iron. When active, IRPs bind to specific parts of the mRNA of genes involved in cellular iron regulation, including transferrin receptor, ferroportin, the iron importer divalent metal transporter 1 (DMT1), and ferritin (Figure 2.3). Specifically, IRPs bind to the 5' (front end) of the mRNA encoding ferritin proteins, which prevents the translation of the mRNA into protein. Conversely, IRPs bind to the 3' (back end) of the mRNA of transferrin receptor – this stabilises this mRNA, which means more transferrin receptor protein is produced.

So, a cell with low iron increases its ability to acquire more iron via transferrin receptor and does not store iron in ferritin; cells with especially high iron demand such as proliferating erythroblasts have very high levels of transferrin receptors. On the other hand, nonproliferating or slowly dividing cells with sufficient iron (e.g. hepatocytes) have inactive IRPs, and make more ferritin to store iron, but less transferrin receptor (Figure 2.3).

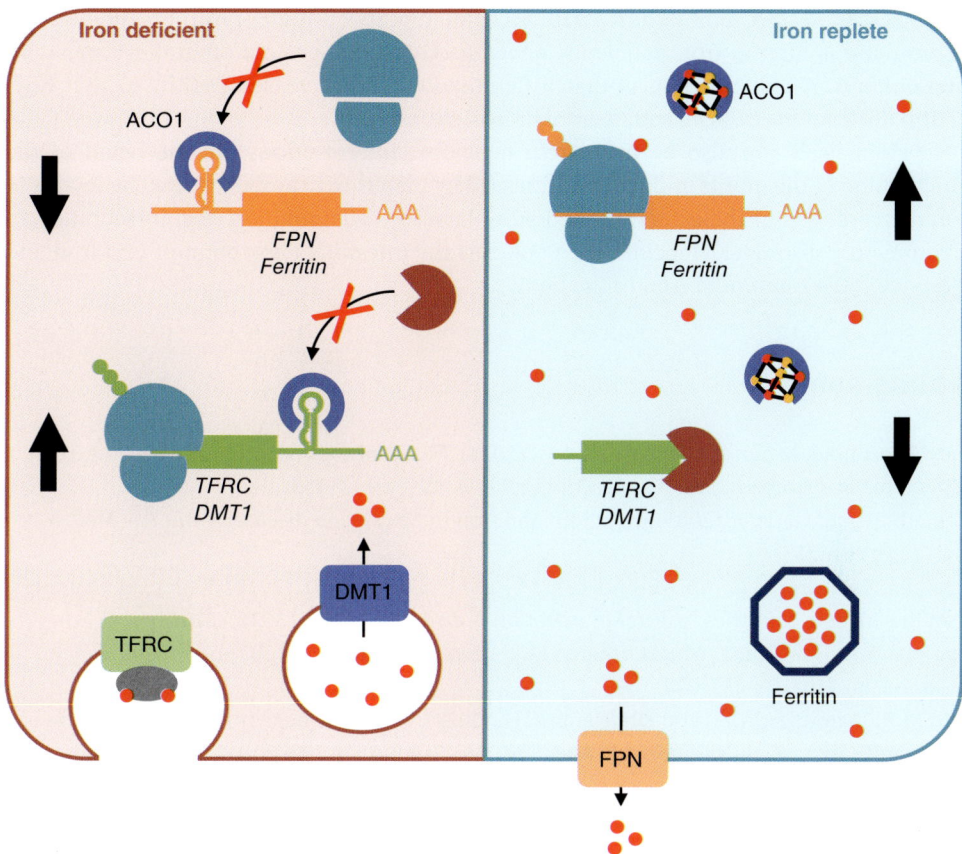

Figure 2.3 The IRP-IRE system. During iron deficient conditions, iron response proteins such as aconitase-1 (ACO1) bind to iron response element (IRE) mRNA structures driving iron uptake. Binding to 5′ IREs in the mRNAs of ferroportin and ferritin blocks translation and results in downregulation. Binding to 3′ IREs in the mRNAs of TFRC and DMT1 prevents degradation by RNAses and allows translations, increasing these proteins. Conversely, under iron replete conditions, ACO1 binding is blocked by a [4Fe-4S] cluster promoting iron sequestration and egress. Ferroportin and ferritin mRNAs with 5′ IREs can be translated whereas TFRC and DMT1 mRNAs with 3′ IREs are degraded by RNAses.

Although both transferrin receptor and ferritin are normally cell-associated (membrane protein and cytosolic protein, respectively), they can also be released into plasma.

Assessing Iron Status – How the Markers Used Relate to Underlying Biology

Usefully, the physiological inputs controlling hepcidin and cellular iron have counterparts in plasma markers measured by clinical biochemistry labs. Transferrin saturation and serum ferritin represent iron availability and iron stores and both are decreased in iron deficiency. Increased soluble transferrin receptor reports on high erythropoietic demand for iron and is high in iron deficiency anaemia. C-reactive protein often correlates with interleukin-6. A complication is that inflammation also increases ferritin so that high ferritin does not necessarily equate to high iron stores.

Hepcidin itself can also be measured; hepcidin concentrations are the result of the combination of the inputs and will be increased by high iron stores, decreased by erythroid iron demand (e.g. in thalassaemia) and stimulated by inflammation (e.g. infection or an inflammatory disorder). Hepcidin then controls the intestinal absorption of oral iron and subsequent distribution of iron in the body.

Bibliography

Galy, B., Conrad, M., and Muckenthaler, M. (2024). Mechanisms controlling cellular and systemic iron homeostasis. *Nat Rev Mol Cell Biol.* 25 (2): 133–155.

Nemeth, E. and Ganz, T. (2023). Hepcidin and iron in health and disease. *Annu Rev Med.* 27 (74): 261–277.

Pasricha, S.R., Armitage, A.E., Prentice, A.M., and Drakesmith, H. (2018). Reducing anaemia in low income countries: control of infection is essential. *BMJ* 1 (362): k3165.

Pasricha, S.R., Tye-Din, J., Muckenthaler, M.U., and Swinkels, D.W. (2021). Iron deficiency. *Lancet* 397 (10270): 233–248.

Teh, M.R., Armitage, A.E., and Drakesmith, H. (2024). Why cells need iron: a compendium of iron utilisation. *Trends Endocrinol Metab* S1043-2760 (24): 00109–00107.

3

Iron and Immunity

Fabiana Busti[1,2] and Domenico Girelli[1,2]

[1] *Department of Medicine, Section of Internal Medicine, University of Verona, Italy*
[2] *Veneto Region Referral Center for Iron Disorders and European Reference Network Center for Rare Hematological Diseases "EuroBloodNet", Verona, Italy*

Introduction

Due to its unique catalytic and oxy-reductive properties, iron is thought to have played a key role in the development of life on the Earth. Bioavailable iron is relatively scarce, and unicellular and multicellular organisms have evolved several strategies to acquire, store and recycle this essential element.

The Battle for Iron and the Concept of 'Nutritional Immunity'

During an infection, a battle for iron occurs between the pathogen and the human host. From one side, microbes secrete various molecules with a high affinity for iron, called siderophores, which are often unique to different bacterial strains. Amongst them are enterobactin, produced by Enterobacteriaceae, and staphyloferrins, produced by *Staphylococcus aureus.*

The host reacts by producing similar iron-binding proteins like lactoferrin, calprotectin and lipocalin-2, known as neutrophil gelatinase-associated lipocalin (NGAL). Under the control of pro-inflammatory cytokines like interleukin-6 (IL-6), the host also produces hepcidin, the liver peptide hormone central to systemic iron homeostasis (reviewed in Chapter 2). This quickly results in hypoferraemia due to the sequestration of iron into mononuclear cells (Figure 3.1). Notably, hepcidin is a small (25 amino acid), cationic peptide folded by four disulphide bounds, structurally analogue to defensins, a family of peptides of innate immunity with direct antimicrobial activity produced by neutrophils and epithelial cells. Hence, hepcidin stands at the crossroads between iron metabolism and immunity by exerting a prevalently *indirect* antimicrobial activity through the subtraction of iron to invading pathogens.

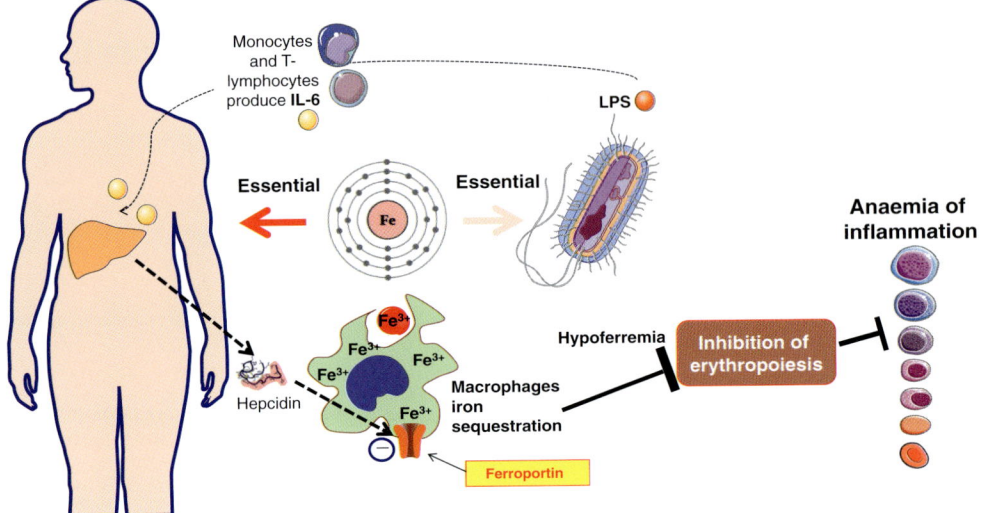

Figure 3.1 Hepcidin has an indirect antimicrobial activity by reducing iron availability to invading pathogens. IL-6, interleukin-6; LPS, lipopolysaccharide.

This mechanism also substantially contributes to the pathogenesis of the anaemia of inflammation, the second commonest cause of anaemia worldwide and the first in hospitalised patients.

Finally, with infections by intracellular pathogens, there is activation of the natural resistance-associated macrophage protein 1 (NRAMP1), a structural analogue to the divalent metal transporter 1 (DMT1). NRAMP1 then leads to iron starvation of the intracellular pathogen by exporting iron from the phagolysosome. The complex multiple mechanisms used by the host to deprive microbes of essential trace minerals (not only iron but also zinc and manganese) are collectively termed 'nutritional immunity'.

Therapeutic Interventions Harnessing Nutritional Immunity

Infections due to multi-drug resistant (MDR) pathogens represent a growing major public health problem, estimated to become one of the leading causes of death worldwide in the next decades. Novel antibiotics are urgently needed to combat such a crisis. An attractive strategy is to target bacterial metal uptake systems through 'Trojan horse' antimicrobials. This class includes antibiotics conjugated with siderophores to ensure uptake by bacterial metal transport systems. Cefiderecol is an FDA-approved, first-in-class metalloantibiotic cephalosporine with activity against MDR Enterobacteriaceae, consisting of a chlorocatechol group that chelates iron. At variance with conventional β-lactams that enter bacteria by passive transport through porin channels, cefiderecol also enters by active transport through the bacteria's iron carrier transport system. This allows the achievement of higher concentration within the bacterial periplasm, as well as stability against β-lactamases. Metalloantibiotics represent an active field of research that may give rise to other useful compounds in the near future.

Iron Status and Susceptibility to Infections

Beyond the synthesis of haemoglobin and oxygen transport, iron is involved in many other vital functions (reviewed in Chapter 1), including mitochondrial energy production and cell proliferation, as several enzymes controlling DNA synthesis and repair are ferroproteins (Figure 3.2). Iron is also essential for human host defences, being a cofactor of iron-dependent, pathogen-eliminating enzymes like myeloperoxidase and nitric oxide synthase. In particular, an efficient B-lymphocyte-driven adaptive immunity to infectious agents or vaccines requires a metabolic burst for antibody synthesis and cell proliferation that may be blunted in conditions of iron deficiency.

The role of iron in the immune response is underscored by a rare disease model due to mutations in the gene encoding for transferrin receptor 1 (*TFRC*), the main protein involved in cellular iron uptake. Contrary to expectations, *TFRC* mutations lead not only to mild anaemia but also to severe childhood infections due to a unique subtype of combined immunodeficiency with functional impairment of either T or B lymphocytes.

Iron Deficiency and Health of Populations

Anaemia, mostly due to iron deficiency, is the most frequent disease and cause of disability worldwide, particularly in areas with high infectious disease burden and in groups that are frequently vaccinated, such as infants, pregnant women and the elderly. Theoretically, routine iron supplementation may not only correct anaemia but also reinforce immune defences against infections. However, the relationships between iron deficiency and infections are far more complex than this simplistic view. For example, it has been demonstrated that iron deficiency confers some protection from malaria in endemic areas. Furthermore, treating anaemia with iron supplementation may favour malaria progression due to parasite tropism for the reticulocytes released during recovery. Thus, in malaria-endemic regions, iron supplementation should be given only on the proviso that concomitant strategies to prevent and treat malaria are implemented.

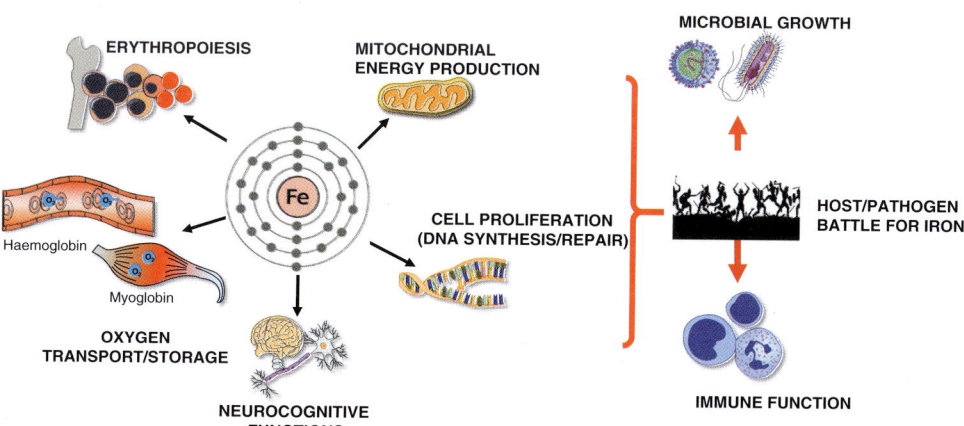

Figure 3.2 Beyond haemoglobin: iron is essential for many vital functions.

Iron Overload and Risk of Infection

Iron overload can also predispose to infection, including sepsis, as recently shown by a Danish population study in carriers of the C282Y genotype associated with haemochromatosis.

Several individual cases of severe infection by *Vibrio vulnificus*, an iron-avid pathogen, have been reported in patients with haemochromatosis. On this basis, guidelines recommend individuals with haemochromatosis avoid wound contact with seawater or eating uncooked seafood especially in subtropical areas where *V. vulnificus* is endemic.

Iron Status and Response to Vaccines

More recently, research has focused on the effect of iron status on vaccine responses. Iron deficiency has been associated with a blunted response to influenza virus vaccination in elderly people. In African infants, anaemia and/or iron deficiency at the time of vaccination have been associated with decreased response to certain vaccines, including diphtheria, pertussis and pneumococcal. Iron supplementation before vaccination has been associated with improved responses, especially to the measles vaccine. Although encouraging, these studies need to be corroborated by large trials before evidence-based recommendations can be implemented in clinical practice.

The dose, route of administration and timing of iron supplementation should be standardised. Nevertheless, the co-occurrence of iron deficiency and risk of infection in fragile populations like infants, pregnant women and the elderly, particularly in disadvantageous areas of the planet, make this issue amongst global health priorities. Figure 3.3 summarises current knowledge on how common iron disorders can influence immune function and susceptibility to infections.

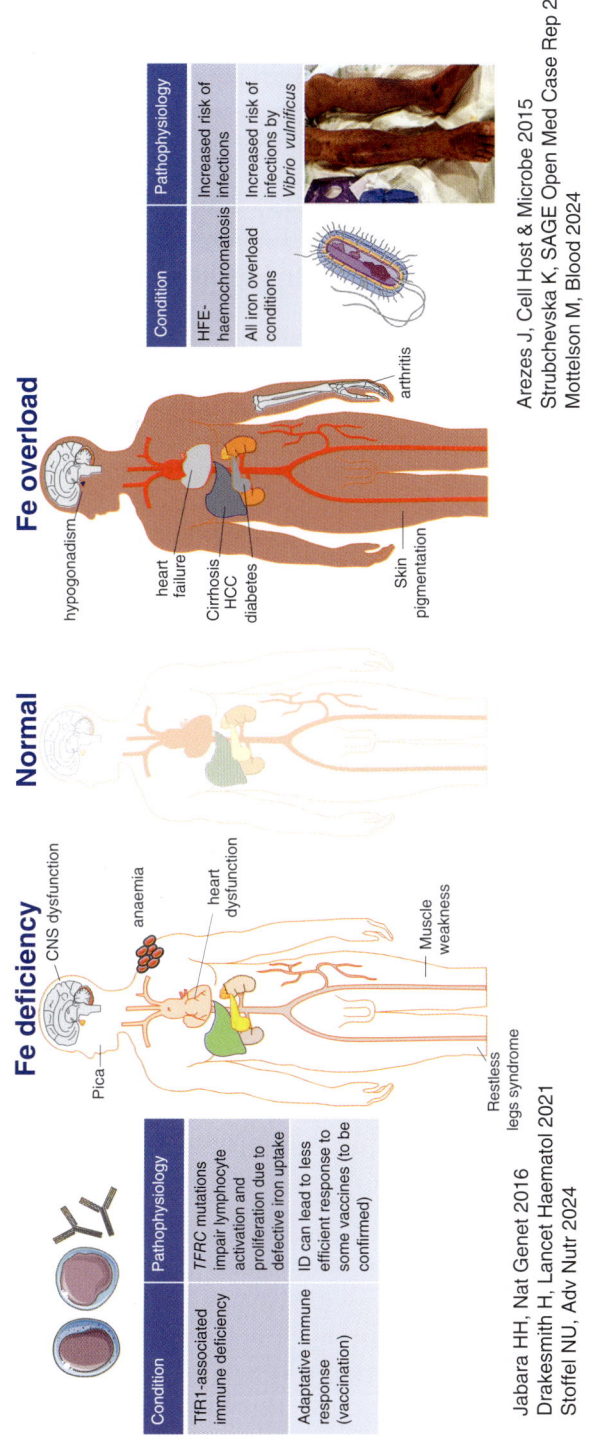

Fe deficiency

Condition	Pathophysiology
TfR1-associated immune deficiency	*TFRC* mutations impair lymphocyte activation and proliferation due to defective iron uptake
Adaptive immune response (vaccination)	ID can lead to less efficient response to some vaccines (to be confirmed)

Jabara HH, Nat Genet 2016
Drakesmith H, Lancet Haematol 2021
Stoffel NU, Adv Nutr 2024

CNS dysfunction
anaemia
heart dysfunction
Pica
Muscle weakness
Restless legs syndrome

Normal

Fe overload

hypogonadism
heart failure
Cirrhosis
HCC
diabetes
Skin pigmentation
arthritis

Condition	Pathophysiology
HFE-haemochromatosis	Increased risk of infections
All iron overload conditions	Increased risk of infections by *Vibrio vulnificus*

Arezes J, Cell Host & Microbe 2015
Strubchevska K, SAGE Open Med Case Rep 2023
Mottelson M, Blood 2024

TfR1: transferrin receptor 1; TFRC: transferrin receptor gene; ID: iron deficiency; CNS: central nervous system; HCC: hepatocellular carcinoma.

Figure 3.3 How common iron disorders can influence immune function and susceptibility to infections. TfR1, transferrin receptor 1; TFRC, transferrin receptor gene; ID, iron deficiency; CNS, central nervous system; HCC, hepatocellular carcinoma (Arezes 2015; Jabara 2016; Drakesmith 2021; Strubchevska et al. 2023; Mottelson 2024; Stoffel 2024). *Source:* Strubchevska et al. (2023)/with permission of SAGE Publications.

Bibliography

Arezes, J., Jung, G., Gabayan, V. et al. (2015). Hepcidin-induced hypoferremia is a critical host defense mechanism against the siderophilic bacterium Vibrio vulnificus. *Cell Host Microbe* 17 (1): 47–57.

Camaschella, C. and Girelli, D. (2020). The changing landscape of iron deficiency. *Mol Aspects Med* 75: 100861.

Drakesmith, H., Pasricha, S.R., Cabantchik, I. et al. (2021). Vaccine efficacy and iron deficiency: an intertwined pair? *Lancet Haematol* 8 (9): e666–e669.

Frei, A., Verderosa, A.D., Elliott, A.G. et al. (2023). Metals to combat antimicrobial resistance. *Nat Rev Chem* 7 (3): 202–224.

Ganz, T. and Nemeth, E. (2024). Hypoferremia of inflammation: innate host defense against infections. *Blood Cells Mol Dis* 104: 102777.

Jabara, H.H., Boyden, S.E., Chou, J. et al. (2016). A missense mutation in TFRC, encoding transferrin receptor 1, causes combined immunodeficiency. *Nat Genet* 48 (1): 74–78.

Mottelson, M., Glenthøj, A., Nordestgaard, B.G. et al. (2024). Iron, hemochromatosis genotypes, and risk of infections: a cohort study of 142188 general population individuals. *Blood* 144 (7): 693–707.

Stoffel, N.U. and Drakesmith, H. (2024). Effects of iron status on adaptive immunity and vaccine efficacy: a review. *Adv Nutr* 15 (6): 100238.

Stoffel, N.U. and Drakesmith, H. (2024). Effects of iron status on adaptive immunity and vaccine efficacy: a review. *Adv Nutr* 15 (6): 100238.

Strubchevska, K., Kozyk, M., and Marijanovich, N. (2023). *SAGE Open Med Case Rep* 11:2050313X231172329.

Teh, M.R., Armitage, A.E., and Drakesmith, H. (2024). Why cells need iron: a compendium of iron utilisation. *Trends Endocrinol Metab*.

Part 2

Iron Deficiency

Part 2a

Assessment and Management of Iron Deficiency

4

Impact of Iron Deficiency on the Individual

Patrick Kyei-Mensah

Department of Haematology, Oxford University Hospitals NHS Foundation Trust, Oxford, UK

Introduction

Iron deficiency, defined as a reduction in total body iron content below normal levels, is the most common nutritional deficiency worldwide and presents as a spectrum of disorders, ranging from its earliest and mildest form, iron depletion, to its late and most advanced form, iron deficiency anaemia (Figure 4.1).

Iron depletion is the state in which body iron stores are diminished but in the presence of normal haemoglobin concentration. It is the earliest phase of iron deficiency. Prussian blue staining of the bone marrow, if it was done, would show absent iron stores. Ferritin levels will start to fall.

Untreated iron depletion may progress to the next stage, characterised by iron-deficient erythropoiesis, resulting in reduced haemoglobin production in individual red cells but not to a degree sufficient to lead to a decrease in the overall haemoglobin concentration of the total erythron mass. Red cell indices (mean cell volume [MCV] and mean cell haemoglobin [MCH]) are reduced. This state is described as non-anaemic iron deficiency and is characterised by depletion of body iron stores, together with measurable and variable reductions in serum iron indices such as ferritin and transferrin saturation (Figure 4.2).

Diagnosis of non-anaemic iron deficiency requires a high index of suspicion (see Table 4.1), requiring scrutiny and evaluation of laboratory parameters such as red cell indices, platelet count and serum iron indices in at-risk groups. Unfortunately, such meticulous attention to laboratory blood results in a patient with normal haemoglobin concentration is uncommon in everyday clinical practice, meaning that, much of the iron-deficiency-associated morbidity burden escapes clinical attention and appropriate corrective therapy.

Iron deficiency anaemia represents the most advanced form and is characterised by absent body iron stores and markedly reduced serum iron indices, in addition to variable reductions in blood haemoglobin concentration.

Iron in Clinical Practice, First Edition. Edited by Sue Pavord and Noemi Roy.
© 2025 John Wiley & Sons Ltd. Published 2025 by John Wiley & Sons Ltd.
Companion website: www.wiley.com/go/medicine5e

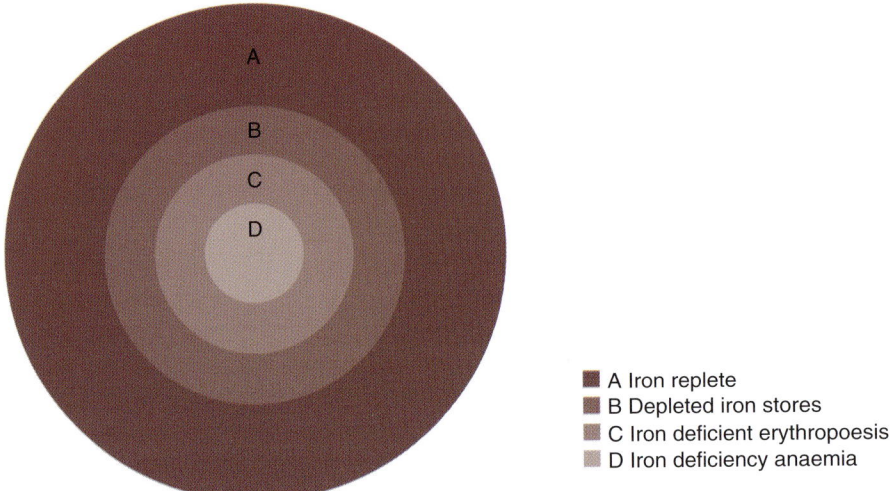

A Iron replete
B Depleted iron stores
C Iron deficient erythropoesis
D Iron deficiency anaemia

Figure 4.1   Progressive stages of iron depletion.

Symptoms and Signs of Iron Deficiency

Because iron is such an essential element for a multitude of body biological functions, including synthesis of haemoglobin and myoglobin, cellular regulation, DNA synthesis, mitochondrial electron transport pathways and many other enzymatic processes, it is not surprising that iron deficiency is associated with a wide array of symptoms with a negative impact on well-being. This is particularly true of tissues with a high cell turnover such as haemopoietic tissue, skin, mucus membranes and hair follicles, which explains the association of iron deficiency of sufficient severity, with symptoms like glossitis, stomatitis and koilonychia. *Plummer–Vinson* syndrome, a condition characterised by dysphagia resulting from oropharyngeal and laryngeal mucosal atrophy, has been described in severe cases of untreated iron deficiency.

Hair loss is another commonly reported symptom and generally accepted to be a complication of severe iron deficiency. However, the evidence for lesser degrees of iron deficiency is, at best, conflicting, perhaps because of the lack of uniformity in how iron deficiency is defined and the presence of uncontrolled confounding factors such as thyroid function status, gonadal hormonal status and presence or absence of other co-existent nutritional deficiencies.

Other reported symptoms of iron deficiency are indicated in Table 4.1.

Impact of Iron Deficiency on Specific At-risk Groups

Though iron deficiency and iron deficiency anaemia can present at any age in both males and females, it is particularly prevalent amongst specific demographic groups where demand for iron is increased. These include infancy and early childhood, pregnancy and the postpartum period, non-pregnant premenopausal women and in regular blood donors.

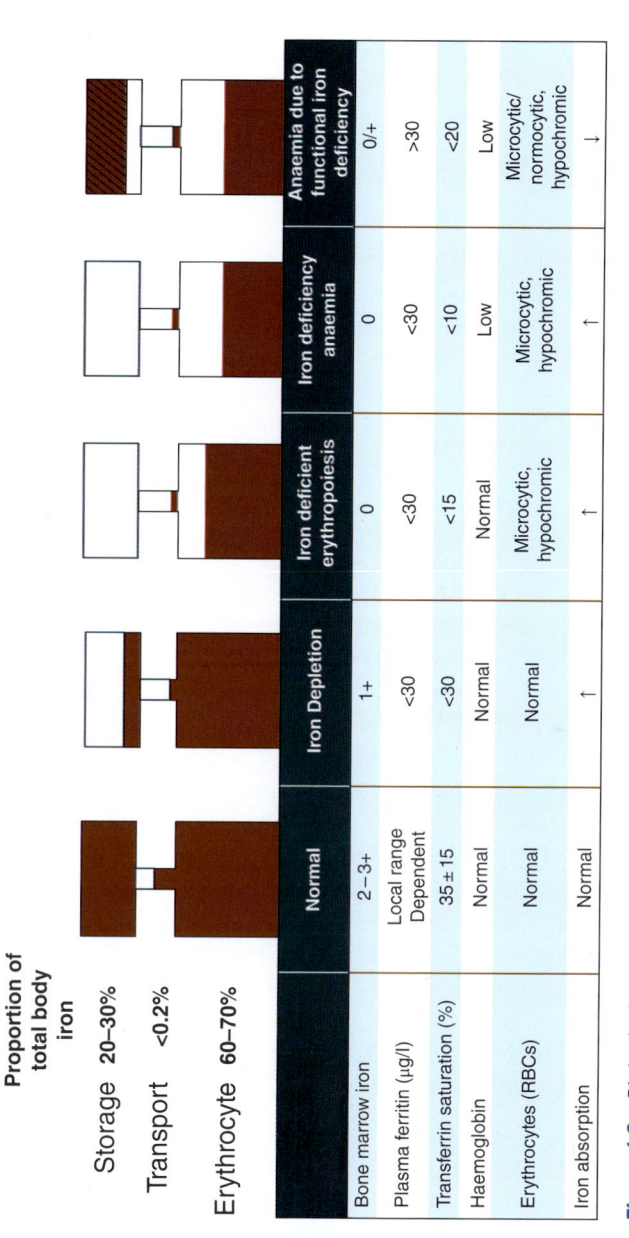

Proportion of total body iron

Storage   20–30%

Transport   <0.2%

Erythrocyte   60–70%

	Normal	Iron Depletion	Iron deficient erythropoiesis	Iron deficiency anaemia	Anaemia due to functional iron deficiency
Bone marrow iron	2–3+	1+	0	0	0/+
Plasma ferritin (µg/l)	Local range Dependent	<30	<30	<30	>30
Transferrin saturation (%)	35 ± 15	<30	<15	<10	<20
Haemoglobin	Normal	Normal	Normal	Low	Low
Erythrocytes (RBCs)	Normal	Normal	Microcytic, hypochromic	Microcytic, hypochromic	Microcytic/ normocytic, hypochromic
Iron absorption	Normal	↑	↑	↑	↓

Figure 4.2 Biological changes through the stages of iron depletion.

Table 4.1 Reported symptoms in patients with iron deficiency with or without anaemia.

System	Symptoms
Skin	Pallor
	Angular cheilosis
	Pruritus
Mucus membranes	Glossitis
	Dysphagia (from oral and laryngopharyngeal mucosal atrophy)
Nails	Koilonychia (spoon nails)
	Brittle nails
Hair	Loss of hair
Neurological	General irritability
	Poor concentration
	Headaches
	Hyperactivity syndromes
	Attention deficit disorders
	Restless legs syndrome (*Ekbom's disease*)
Neuropsychiatric	Anxiety
	Mental depression
General	Tiredness
	Lethargy
	Muscle weakness
	Diminished work performance
	Pica

Pregnancy, Parturition and Lactation

Pregnancy, parturition and lactation impose very heavy iron demands on the female body. It is estimated that in a normal pregnancy, the average total amount of iron diverted from mother to fetus, the amount lost during delivery and through lactation, adds up to over 1000 mg. Cumulative iron losses through menstrual bleeding means most women start pregnancy with varying degrees of iron deficiency, with up to 85% of all women worldwide affected.

This has been associated with a high incidence of maternal illness and poor pregnancy outcomes and fetal and neonatal morbidity (Chapter 13).

Paediatric Population

Though iron is one of the most important dietary nutrients, iron deficiency is one of the most prevalent nutritional deficiencies in children, with an estimated 300 million children reported to have been affected worldwide, in the year 2011. Infants and young children are at particular risk of iron deficiency because of the increased iron requirements needed to support a rapidly expanding body and red cell mass.

As iron plays a crucial role in the development of a growing child's brain, and consequently in the moulding of mental capacity and psychological development, it is not surprising that infants and children with iron deficiency, with or without anaemia, present with neurological symptoms of general irritability, delayed physical and behavioural development, poor attention span and various hyperactivity syndromes. Other reported sequelae of iron deficiency in this age group include mild to moderate degrees of cognitive impairment, reduced emotional responsiveness and learning disabilities.

Non-pregnant Premenopausal Women

Iron deficiency and iron deficiency anaemia are very common conditions in non-pregnant premenopausal women, largely as a consequence of cumulative iron losses through monthly menstruation. It is estimated that about one-fifth (20%) of all women under the age of 50 years have one form of iron deficiency or the other. Symptoms reported in this group of patients include excessive fatigue, irritability, tiredness, excessive hair loss and a reduced quality of life.

Individuals from Resource-poor Settings

Iron deficiency is more prevalent in low and middle income countries due to poorer nutrition and presence of parasitic infections such as hookworm.

Other Clinical Situations Associated with Iron Deficiency

Gastrointestinal Bleeding

In post-menopausal women and adult men, iron deficiency anaemia is often the presenting feature of chronic lower intestinal bleeding, such as benign colonic polyps, malignancies and angiodysplasia. Iron deficiency from occult upper gastrointestinal bleeding is also a common presentation in patients with acid peptic disorders, including gastric and duodenal ulcers, hiatus hernia, oesophagitis and gastritis induced by corticosteroids, non-steroidal anti-inflammatory drug induced gastritis, alcohol and antiplatelet agents.

Heart Failure

Iron deficiency (defined as either ferritin <100 mcg/L or <300 mcg/L with a transferrin saturation of <20%) is common in patients with heart failure, affecting up to 59% of this patient cohort.

Affected patients present with reduced exercise tolerance and capacity, reduction in physical activity and performance, increased risk of hospitalisation and hospital readmissions, reduced quality of life and higher mortality rates compared to iron replete patients with equivalent degrees of cardiac dysfunction.

Chronic Obstructive Airway Disease

Iron deficiency has been found to be more prevalent in patients with chronic obstructive airway disease (COPD) than in patients without the condition. Between a third and half of patients with COPD have iron deficiency, which has a negative impact on prognosis and disease progression.

Renal Disease

About 50% of patients with chronic kidney disease (CKD) have iron deficiency, with a significant proportion also with concurrent anaemia. As with other anaemias, iron deficiency anaemia in CKD is associated with an increased risk of morbidity and mortality.

Conclusion

Given the high prevalence of both non-anaemic iron depletion and iron deficiency anaemia, and the significant impact of these on the individual, health care workers must maintain a high index of suspicion, so that these states do not go undiagnosed.

Bibliography

Benson, C.S., Shah, A., Frise, M.C., and Frise, C.J. (2021). Iron deficiency anaemia in pregnancy: a contemporary review. *2021 Jun;14(2):67-76. Obstet Med* 14 (2): 67–76. https://doi.org/10.1177/1753495X20932426.

J D Haas, T Brownlie Iron deficiency and reduced work capacity: a critical review of the research to determine a causal relationship. *J Nutr* 2001; 131(2S-2):676S-688S. https://doi.org/10.1093/jn/131.2.676S

Sawada, T. and Konomi, Y.K. (2014). Iron deficiency anaemia is associated with anger and fatigue in young Japanese women. *Biol Trace Elem Res* 159 (1–3): 22–31.

Schrage, B., Rubsamen, N., Schulz, A. et al. (2020). Iron deficiency is a common disorder in general population and independently predicts all-cause mortality: results from the Gutenberg Health Study. *Clin Res Cardiol* 109 (11): 1352–1357. https://doi.org/10.1007/s00392-020-01631-y.

Soppi, E.T. (2018). Iron deficiency without anaemia – a clinical challenge. *Clin Case Rep* 6: 1082–1086.

Weyland, A.C., Chaitoff, A., and Freed, G.L. (2023). Prevalence of iron deficiency and iron deficiency anaemia in US females aged 12-21 years, 2003-2020. *JAMA* 329 (24): 2191–2193.

5

Assessment of Iron Deficiency

Hanke L. Matlung[1] and Dorine W. Swinkels[2,3]

[1] Sanquin Research and Landsteiner Laboratory, Department of Molecular Hematology, Amsterdam, the Netherlands
[2] Sanquin Blood Bank, Amsterdam, the Netherlands
[3] Department of Laboratory Medicine, Radboud University Medical Center, Nijmegen, the Netherlands

Introduction

Accurate assessment of body iron status is difficult; there is no one test, or combination of tests, that reliably quantifies available iron in all clinical conditions. In this vacuum, serum ferritin is currently considered the gold standard, as a low level is specific to iron deficiency (ID), but like all available tests, this too has its limitations.

Definitions

ID is classified as absolute ID in cases when total body iron stores are insufficient to meet the iron demand. In patients with inflammation, total body iron levels are generally adequate but iron is distributed out of the circulation to the macrophages of the reticuloendothelial system (RES), causing functional ID or anaemia of chronic disease (Figure 5.1). ID anaemia (IDA) is defined as low Hb or haematocrit and is associated with microcytic and hypochromic red blood cells (RBC) and low RBC count.

Ferritin Thresholds

The diagnosis for ID and IDA and their severity is based on assessment of specific haematological parameters as well as biomarkers for iron (Figure 5.2, Table 5.1). Ferritin levels in serum or plasma reflect total-body iron stores, where World Health Organisation (WHO) defined that levels below 15 µg/L are a good predictor for absent iron in bone marrow and ID in children >5 years, adolescents and adults, although suggestions have been made to increase the ferritin cutoff value for ID to 30 µg/L. Variety in worldwide ferritin decision

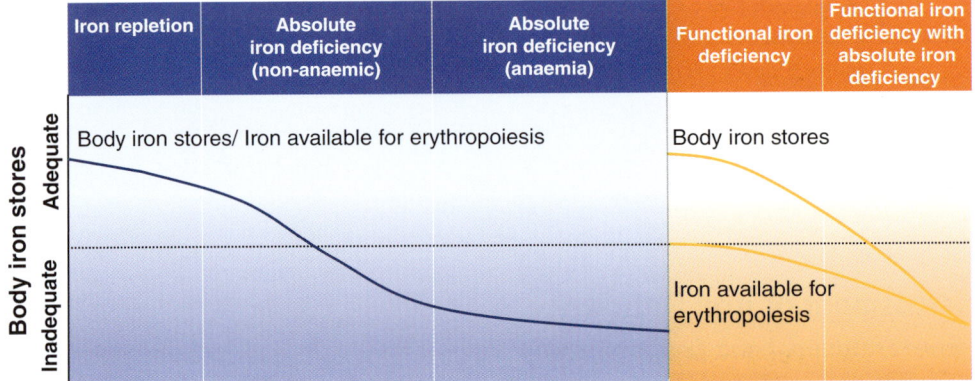

Figure 5.1 Adequacy of body iron stores in various forms of ID and IDA. *Source:* Adapted from Pasricha et al. (2021) (top of Figure 3).

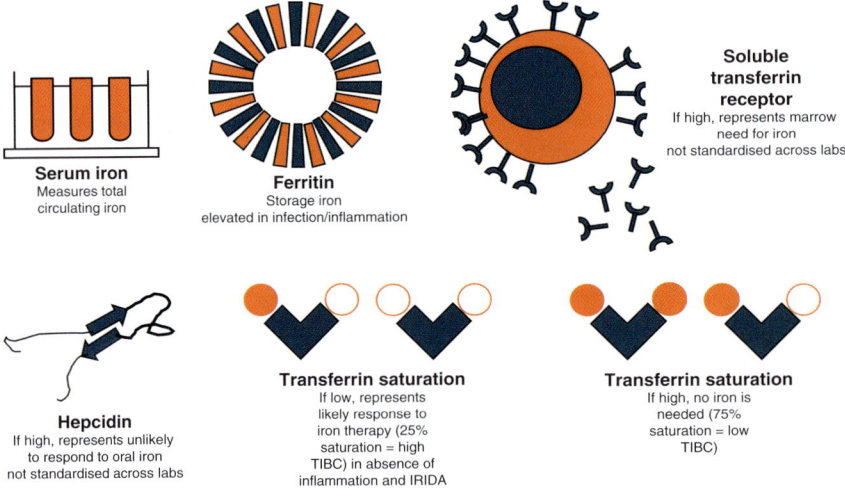

Figure 5.2 Biomarkers in diagnosis and monitoring of ID. In the absence of inflammation, patients with low transferrin saturation (TSAT) are likely to respond well to oral or intravenous iron with the exception of patients diagnosed with iron refractory iron deficiency anaemia (IRIDA). TIBC, total iron binding capacity or transferrin.

limits for IDA and ID can be attributed to various forms of heterogeneity and bias in studies, including shortcomings in the definition of the normal population and, more importantly, lack of standardisation of ferritin assays. To address the latter, the WHO initiated development of ferritin reference materials more than three decades ago. However, these preparations lack traceability to each other. Since most used ferritin assays claim traceability to three different generations of WHO reference materials, it resulted in substantial between-assay variation. Moreover, recent studies suggest WHO reference materials may not be optimally commutable, i.e. may show other between-method differences than native human samples, precluding standardisation. Altogether this suboptimal harmonisation

Table 5.1 Laboratory tests for ID in adults.

Iron status Test	ID	Functional ID	ID anaemia	Anaemia of chronic disease	ID' anaemia and anaemia of chronic disease	IRIDA	Reference interval
Conventional							
Iron (μmol/L)	Low	Low–normal	Low	Low	Low	Low	13–36
Transferrin (g/L)/TIBC (μmol/L)	High	Normal	High	Low	Variable	High	2.0–3.6 / 45–78
TSAT (%)	<15–20[a]	<15–20[a]	<15[a]	<15–20[a]	<15–20[a]	<10	15–45
Ferritin (μg/L)	<15[a]	<70[a]	<15[a]	<70[a]	<70[a]	Variable	M: 15–200[a] / F: 15–150[a]
Hb (g/dL) Men/women	Normal	Normal	Low	Low	Low	Low	>13/ >12
MCV (fL)	Normal	Normal	<80	Low–normal	Low	Low	80–95
Bone marrow iron	Negative	Variable	Negative	Positive	Positive	Positive	Positive
Emerging							
Hepcidin	Low	High	Very low	High–low	High–low	High for TSAT	Varies[a]
sTfR (mg/L)	High	High	High	Low–normal	Variable	High	Varies[a]
sTfR /log ferritin	NA	NA	>2[a]	<1[a]	>2[a]	NA	Varies[a]
Reticulocyte HbC(pg)	<28[a]	<29[a]	Low	Low–normal	Low	Low	30.2–35.9[a]

NA, not available; TIBC, total iron binding capacity; TSAT, transferrin saturation; sTfR, soluble transferrin receptors.

[a] Vary with the methodology or calibration used.

Source: Swinkels (2023)/with permission of Elsevier.

and standardisation between commercial ferritin assays results in considerable interassay variation and impacts on clinical decision-making based on ferritin concentrations. Until future efforts address these aspects, thresholds for ferritin concentration defining ID and IDA will remain to some extent arbitrary.

Inflammation and Liver Disease

The use of ferritin to diagnose ID in a setting of inflammation is hampered by the fact that ferritin is also an acute phase protein. Strategies have been developed to correct for this, by making use of regression equations correlating inflammatory markers to ferritin levels or by arbitrarily raising the threshold of ferritin to 70 µg/L in children >5 years and adults when inflammation is apparent. Increased ferritin levels are further caused by liver disease, in particular nonalcoholic fatty liver disease, metabolic syndrome or malignancy. Thereby, for a certain degree of body iron levels, it is suggested that ferritin levels are higher in conditions where iron is preferentially distributed in reticuloendothelial system (RES) macrophages (Kupffer cells and in spleen), compared to iron mostly stored in parenchymal cells (such as hepatocytes).

Additional Biomarkers

As the amount of iron available for erythropoiesis cannot be accurately assessed by ferritin levels alone, and serum iron concentration is reduced in ID as well as inflammation, combination with additional parameters provides a better (functional) indication to identify adequacy of iron supply for erythropoiesis. These include transferrin saturation (TSAT), soluble or serum transferrin receptor (sTfR), haemoglobin content of reticulocytes (Ret HbC) and the percentage of hypochromic erythrocytes (%HypoEry) (Figure 5.2, Table 5.1). TSAT reflects both serum concentrations of iron and transferrin-binding capacity. TSATs below 15% defines inadequate iron supply for production of haemoglobin and RBC in both absolute and functional ID in adults. The expression of cellular TfR, predominantly in erythroid precursor cells, is regulated by the amount of available iron, where its mRNA is stabilised in case of limiting iron availability. Therefore, sTfR levels in plasma reflect whether iron meets erythropoeitic needs. In clinical practice, the sTfR/log ferritin ratio turned out a useful predictive index for iron stores in bone marrow, especially in inflammatory conditions. Under these circumstances, cellular TfR levels remain mostly normal, making sTfR levels useful in distinguishing between inflammatory conditions (i.e. anaemia of chronic disease) and ID, both associated with low serum iron and low TSAT (Table 5.1). In practice, utility of sTfR is limited, due to low clinical availability and high interassay variability, which could be relieved by the worldwide implementation of the WHO reference material.

Red Cell Indices

Progression of ID induces changes in red cell indices (Figure 5.3), as red cells become increasingly microcytic (low MCV) and hypochromic (low MCH). Indices such as Ret HbC can be measured on several automated haematology analysers, and this parameter

Marker \ Stage	Depleted iron store	Iron deficiency, normal Hb	Iron deficiency anaemia
Bone marrow,	————————————————————————————→		
Ferritin	————————————————————————————→		
Hepcidin	————————————————————————————→		
TSAT		————————————————————→	
sTfR		————————————————————→	
Ret HbC		————————————————————→	
%HypoEry		————————————————————→	
Hb, MCV/MCH			——————————————→

Figure 5.3 Alterations in biochemical and haematological parameters at different stages of ID and IDA. *Source:* Swinkels (2023)/with permission of Elsevier.

reflects recent (3–4 days before testing) iron available for erythropoiesis. The percentage of RBCs that are hypochromic (%HypoEry) represents iron restriction for the bone marrow 2–3 months preceding analysis. Both parameters are useful in the assessment of response to iron treatment and provide insight in whether the iron-restricted erythropoiesis is due to absolute ID or the consequence of ACD, since the latter condition generally results in the formation of normocytic and normochromic RBCs.

Hepcidin Levels

Finally, hepcidin concentrations reflect systemic status of iron homeostasis, and measurement might help in the distinction between absolute and functional ID. Hepcidin levels are decreased under hypoxic conditions, increased erythropoietic activity and reduced levels of circulating and stored iron. Inflammation and infection lead to an increase in hepcidin levels, a way of the body to sequester iron within the RES, reducing iron in the circulation. In the presence of severe anaemia, however, hepcidin levels can be normal or even decreased despite inflammation, perhaps a protective effect to reduce life-threatening consequences of the anaemia itself. Low hepcidin levels are predictive for responsiveness to iron treatment and as such allow personalisation of iron supplementation routes.

Several iron disorders lead to dysregulation of hepcidin production, such as seen in Iron Refractory Iron Deficiency Anaemia (IRIDA). IRIDA is a consequence of variants in the *TMPRSS6* gene and results in inappropriately high hepcidin levels relative to transferrin-bound iron in circulation. The TSAT/hepcidin ratio has been proven useful in the diagnosis of these patients. To be able to internationally use hepcidin measurements in diagnostic and research settings, worldwide standardisation is a necessary step, that requires implementation of the recently developed reference material.

Conclusion

In summary, a low serum ferritin concentration is a sensitive indicator of ID uncomplicated by other concurrent diseases. Several other conventional and emerging iron and haematological parameters contribute and complement each other to diagnose and characterise the severity of ID and its functional consequences in haemoglobin synthesis in the individual patient with and without comorbidities.

Bibliography

Braga, F., Pasqualetti, S., Frusciante, E. et al. (2022). Harmonization status of serum ferritin measurements and implications for use as marker of iron-related disorders. *Clin Chem.* 68 (9): 1202–1210.

Diepeveen, L.E., Laarakkers, C.M.M., Martos, G. et al. (2019). Provisional standardization of hepcidin assays: creating a traceability chain with a primary reference material, candidate reference method and a commutable secondary reference material. *Clin Chem Lab Med.* 57 (6): 864–872. https://doi.org/10.1515/cclm-2018-0783.

Lyle, A.N., Budd, J.R., Kennerley, V.M. et al. (2023). Assessment of WHO 07/202 reference material and human serum pools for commutability and for the potential to reduce variability among soluble transferrin receptor assays. *Clin Chem Lab Med.* 61 (10): 1719–1729. https://doi.org/10.1515/cclm-2022-1198.

Pasricha, S.R., Tye-Din, J., Muckenthaler, M.U., Swinkels, D.W. (2021). Iron deficiency. *Lancet* 397 (10270): 233–248.

Swinkels, D.W. (2023). Iron metabolism, Chapter 40. In: *Tietz Textbook of Clinical Chemistry and Molecular Diagnostics*, 7e (ed. N. Rifai, A.R. Horvath, and C. Wittwer). Louis (MO): Elsevier Saunders.

Swinkels, D.W., van Schrojenstein Lantman, M., Matlung, H.L., Weykamp, C., Thelen, M. (2024). Equivalence in clinical assessment of iron status requires ferritin assay standardisation before harmonisation of ferritin reference intervals. *Lancet Haematol.* 11 (10): e721..

Truong, J., Naveed, K., Beriault, D. et al. (2024). The origin of ferritin reference intervals: a systematic review. *Lancet Haematol.* 11: E530–E539.

WHO guideline on haemoglobin cutoffs to define anaemia in individuals and populations (2024). https://iris.who.int/bitstream/handle/10665/376196/9789240088542-eng.pdf?sequence=1

WHO guideline on use of ferritin concentrations to assess iron status in individuals and populations (2020). https://www.who.int/publications/i/item/9789240000124

6

Available Treatments for Iron Deficiency

Paolo Polzella

Department of Haematology, Oxford University Hospitals NHS Foundation Trust, Oxford, UK

Introduction

Iron replacement therapies are widely used in clinical practice to correct iron deficiency, which remains one of the most common causes of anaemia worldwide. Available treatments include oral and intravenous (IV) formulations, and all aim to replenish iron stores, thereby improving haemoglobin levels and oxygen transport. Oral supplements are used in most cases of iron deficiency, but IV iron plays an important role in patients who cannot tolerate oral iron supplements or when rapid iron replenishment is required. The treatments discussed here apply to people with iron deficiency with or without anaemia, as non-anaemic iron depletion is also a significant concern.

Oral Iron Supplementation

Oral iron supplements are the first line of treatment for iron deficiency and are widely used because of their low cost effectiveness and ease of administration. They should be started as soon as the diagnosis is made and in parallel with investigations to determine the cause of the iron deficiency.

Oral iron preparations in common use are listed in Table 6.1. Ferrous fumarate and ferrous sulphate are the preferred preparations, as they provide the ideal dose for absorption and efficacy. Ferrous gluconate contains less elemental iron and is helpful for individuals who have experienced gastrointestinal disturbance with higher strength formulations.

Administration of Oral Iron

Absorption of iron salts is impaired by food, so it is recommended that oral iron supplements be taken at least one hour before meals and drinks, preferably before breakfast when

Iron in Clinical Practice, First Edition. Edited by Sue Pavord and Noemi Roy.
© 2025 John Wiley & Sons Ltd. Published 2025 by John Wiley & Sons Ltd.
Companion website: www.wiley.com/go/medicine5e

Table 6.1 Commonly used oral iron supplements.

Formulation	Preparation	Dose	Elemental iron
Ferrous sulphate	Tablet	200 mg	65 mg
	MR tablet	325 mg	105 mg
	MR capsule	150 mg	48 mg
Ferrous sulphate and ascorbic acid	MR tablet	325 mg	105 mg
Ferrous sulphate and folic acid	MR tablet	325 mg	105 mg
Ferrous fumarate	Tablet	210 mg	69 mg
	Tablet	322 mg	106 mg
	Capsule	305 mg	100 mg
	Liquid	140 mg/5 ml	45 mg/5 ml
Ferrous fumarate and folic acid	Tablet	322 mg	106 mg
Ferrous gluconate	Tablet	300 mg	37 mg
Ferric maltol	Tablet	30 mg	30 mg
Sodium feredetate	Liquid	190 mg/5 ml	27.5 mg/5 ml

MR = modified release dosage.

hepcidin levels are lowest. Notably, tannins in tea completely chelate iron in the gut and prevent absorption, as does the calcium in milk.

Contrary to previous advice to give iron three times a day. Patients should receive oral iron no more than once daily (40–80 mg elemental iron), and for patients with intolerance, such as gastrointestinal upset, the dose or frequency can be titrated downwards. Alternate-day dosing has been shown to provide best absorption, i.e. the functional value of each tablet is optimised. Daily dosing provides slightly higher cumulative iron intake and may be more appropriate when time is limited, such as preoperatively or in pregnancy.

The key to effective use of oral iron is patient counselling. Taken correctly, for optimal absorption, it reduces side effects and has been shown to improve tolerance and compliance. This aspect of management is often forgotten, leading to failure of response and need for IV iron. Joint decision-making between the healthcare provider and the iron-deficient individual is essential to improve compliance (Table 6.2).

Intravenous Iron Therapy

Intravenous (IV) iron replacement therapy is required for iron deficiency in the context of chronic inflammation, where hepcidin levels are elevated and iron absorption impaired. It may also be needed for individuals who cannot tolerate oral iron supplements or where rapid iron replenishment is required, such as in the preoperative setting. IV iron replacement therapy replenishes iron stores more rapidly, but the eventual haemoglobin response is similar to oral iron, so careful assessment is required when prescribing IV iron.

Table 6.2 Administration of oral iron.

Questions for administration	Recommendation	Reason
How much	40–80 mg	Provides optimal absorption
How often	Daily or alternate days	Provides optimal absorption
What with	Water or freshly squeezed orange juice	Vitamin C enhances iron absorption
When	Early morning	Hepcidin levels are lowest
With or without food	One hour before food and drink	To avoid factors that inhibit absorption, such as calcium and tannins
What to avoid	Avoid concomitant medications including multivitamins	Calcium and other metals inhibit absorption

Table 6.3 Intravenous iron formulations in common use.

Formulation	Iron dose	Min infusion	Test dose
Ferric carboxymaltose	Max single dose 20 mg/kg, max 1000 mg	15 min	No
Iron sucrose	200 mg per injection	30 min	Yes
Ferric derisomaltose	Max single dose 20 mg/kg	30 min	No
Iron dextran	Max single dose 20 mg/kg	4–6 h	Yes

Several IV iron formulations are available (Table 6.3), including ferric carboxymaltose and ferric derisomaltose, which contain iron inside a carbohydrate shell designed for uptake by reticuloendothelial macrophages, with subsequent gradual release of iron over time.

In general, the current IV iron preparations are considered to be very safe, with a low risk of serious adverse reactions, as distinct from the historic issues seen with older products such as high-molecular-weight iron dextran, which was not infrequently associated with anaphylactic reactions. Nonetheless, current practice still dictates that IV iron should only be given in clinical environments where resuscitation equipment and expertise are available.

All formulations provide a higher iron load than oral iron, although they are more costly and although adverse effects are unusual, they must be discussed with patients when consent is obtained.

Potential Adverse Effects of Intravenous Iron

Hypersensitivity reactions (including anaphylactic or anaphylactoid reactions) may occur and may vary between formulations, although the incidence is extremely low at around

1:10,000 with the newer preparations. The pathophysiology driving the hypersensitivity reactions is not well understood, although the small amounts of labile iron present have been suggested as a possible cause of drug reactions. If anaphylactic reactions occur, patients should be treated according to the local anaphylaxis protocol with intramuscular adrenaline. Further doses of intravenous iron should be avoided.

Less severe infusion reactions, thought to be associated with free or labile iron release in the circulation, are relatively common and may be seen in 0.5–1% of infusions. These are typically associated with flushing of the face and/or neck and short-lived atypical chest or shoulder pain; these reactions are also known as nontransferrin-bound iron (NTBI) or 'Fishbane' reactions.

Other adverse reactions include hypophosphataemia (see Chapter 10). This has been described with all IV iron formulations but is more likely to occur after ferric carboxymaltose. In the United Kingdom, hypophosphataemia has been the focus of a 2020 medicines safety update from the Medicines and Healthcare products regulatory agency (MHRA), which recommends monitoring serum phosphate levels in patients receiving repeated infusions of ferric carboxymaltose, as cases of hypophosphataemic osteomalacia have been described.

IV iron is contraindicated in pregnant women during the first trimester of pregnancy, where free iron could potentially be toxic to trophoblastic membranes. It should also not be given to patients with active bacteraemia, to avoid enhancing proliferation of pathogens.

IV iron extravasation may result in long-term skin staining, and this risk should be discussed with patients as part of the consent process. The cannula must be well sited, and any localised pain must be reported immediately.

The formulations listed in Table 6.3 are all viable options, although there are differences that may lead a clinician to use one over another. Ferric carboxymaltose and ferric derisomaltose both allow higher doses of iron to be administered in one sitting, making them suitable for rapid correction of iron deficiency. This also circumnavigates compliance difficulties, and their low immunogenicity enables administration in an outpatient setting. Iron sucrose requires multiple doses to achieve complete iron replacement, depending on the underlying cause of iron deficiency and the patient's iron levels.

Individualising Treatment

The choice of supplement, whether oral or IV, depends on the patient's needs and underlying health conditions as well as local protocols and/or formularies. Oral iron supplements are preferred for patients with absolute iron deficiency and low serum ferritin. Those with functional iron deficiency require IV iron due to impaired oral iron absorption. Healthcare professionals providing iron replacement therapy should monitor response to treatment to ensure optimal outcomes and plan further treatment if required. Monitoring usually takes the form of checking Hb 4–6 weeks after treatment has been started, to ensure there is a response, however checking a reticulocyte count after 2 weeks should give an early indication of response. Treatment should be continued for about 3 months to ensure that iron stores are replete. If the cause of the iron deficiency (eg menorrhagia) has not been addressed, assessing for further iron deficiency in future will be needed.

Bibliography

Auerbach, M., Gafter-Gvili, A., and Macdougall, I.C. (2020). Intravenous iron: a framework for changing the management of iron deficiency. *Lancet Haematol* 7 (4): e342–e350.

Dave, C.V., Brittenham, G.M., Carson, J.L., and Setoguchi, S. (2022). Risks for anaphylaxis with intravenous iron formulations: a retrospective cohort study. *Ann Intern Med* 175 (5): 656–664.

Kennedy, N.A., Achebe, M.M., Biggar, P. et al. (2023). A systematic literature review and meta-analysis of the incidence of serious or severe hypersensitivity reactions after administration of ferric derisomaltose or ferric carboxymaltose. *Int J Clin Pharm* 45: 604–612.

Snook, J., Bhala, N., Beales, I.L.P. et al. (2021). British Society of Gastroenterology guidelines for the management of iron deficiency anaemia in adults. *Gut* 70 (11): 2030–2051.

WHO (2021). *The Urgent Need to Implement Patient Blood Management: Policy Brief*. WHO.

Zoller, H., Schaefer, B., and Glodny, B. (2017). Iron-induced hypophosphatemia: an emerging complication. *Curr Opin Nephrol Hypertens* 26 (4): 266–275.

Part 2b

**Causes, Impact, Management and Prevention of
Iron Deficiency in Clinical Specialties**

7

Iron Deficiency in Primary Care

David McCartney

School of Medicine and Biomedical Sciences, Medical Sciences Division, University of Oxford Academic Centre, John Radcliffe Hospital, Oxford, UK

Introduction

Iron deficiency (ID) is common in primary care and can be easily missed as the symptoms are often vague, nonspecific, and overlap with those related to other common presentations. A low threshold for suspecting ID is therefore required. This chapter discusses the recognition of ID in primary care, describing the wide-ranging symptoms, outlines some important and common causes of ID and suggests an approach to investigation based on age.

Presentation of Iron Deficiency in Primary Care

The symptoms of ID are wide ranging and inconsistent but may include fatigue, low energy, reduced exercise tolerance, poor concentration and restless legs syndrome (RLS). Symptoms can impact significantly on daily functions with reduced cognitive function and decreased work productivity and efficiency. As iron plays a critical role in the immune system, individuals with ID may also be more susceptible to infection. The potential societal impacts of ID are significant.

Although there may often be no signs of ID on clinical examination, angular cheilitis, atrophic glossitis or koilonychia may be present (Figure 7.1).

ID anaemia is often also identified incidentally during routine blood tests for other indications or presentations and is occasionally identified via the blood donation process where potential donors are found to be unable to donate due to anaemia and subsequently present to primary care for follow up.

Iron in Clinical Practice, First Edition. Edited by Sue Pavord and Noemi Roy.
© 2025 John Wiley & Sons Ltd. Published 2025 by John Wiley & Sons Ltd.
Companion website: www.wiley.com/go/medicine5e

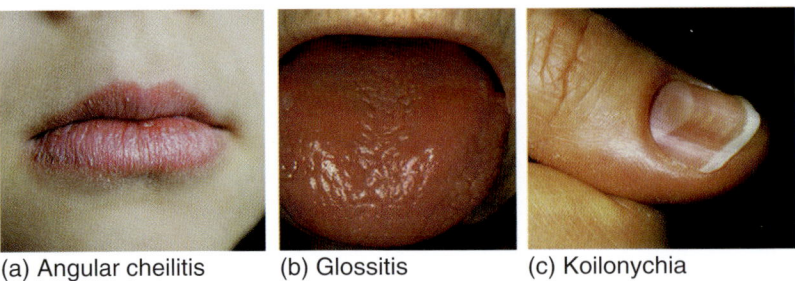

(a) Angular cheilitis   (b) Glossitis   (c) Koilonychia

Figure 7.1 Clinical signs of iron deficiency: angular cheilitis, glossitis and koilonychia. *Sources:* (a) Luci/Adobe Stock; (b) Epomedicine / https://epomedicine.com/clinical-medicine/hematological-signs-angular-stomatitis-and-atrophic-glossitis. (c) National Health Service / https://www.nhs.uk/conditions/nail-problems / Public domain.

The Main Causes of Iron Deficiency in Primary Care

Table 7.1 lists the common causes of ID seen in primary care.

It is also important to consider the causes of ID according to age and sex.

Pre-menopausal Women

By far the most common group presenting to primary care with ID is pre-menopausal women. Pregnancy, miscarriage and menorrhagia are common causes, but often it is simply due to the combination of regular menstruation and inadequate dietary intake. Coeliac disease is found in 3–5% of these cases and needs to be excluded.

Table 7.1 Causes of iron deficiency presenting in primary care.

Inadequate dietary intake	Vegan or vegetarian diet
	Malnutrition
Malabsorption	Coeliac disease
	Helicobacter pylori infection
	Medication related (e.g. proton pump inhibitors)
	Bariatric surgery
	Dietary causes of poor absorption (e.g. excessive tannins in tea and coffee)
Increased blood loss	Regular menstruation
	Gastrointestinal tract pathology (e.g. colorectal malignancy and gastric ulceration)
	Frequent blood donation
Increased iron requirement	Pregnancy
	Breast feeding

Post-menopausal Women and Men

In around one-third of men and post-menopausal women presenting with ID anaemia, an underlying pathological cause is found. This is most commonly identified in the gastrointestinal tract, and a low threshold for further investigation for the cause of ID in these individuals is required to avoid missing potential serious diagnoses, such as a colorectal malignancy.

Older Adults

Anaemia is common in older adults with and without multimorbidity, and the identification of the cause of anaemia may be less straightforward. Where ID is suspected or confirmed, identifying the underlying cause may be more complex, with multiple contributing factors. These may include poor dietary intake, poor gastrointestinal absorption (due to polypharmacy), adverse effects of medication causing occult gastrointestinal blood loss (for example, due to antiplatelets) or gastrointestinal malignancy.

It is worth noting that several chronic diseases commonly managed in primary care can also predispose to both absolute and functional ID, including chronic kidney disease (CKD) and heart failure. This is discussed in more detail in Chapters 10 and 11.

The Diagnosis of Iron Deficiency in Primary Care

Haemoglobin

A microcytic anaemia (with low mean cell volume) with hypochromic cells is consistent with ID anaemia, though it can also be caused by thalassaemia trait and chronic inflammatory conditions. A normocytic anaemia does not exclude ID as a cause of anaemia and iron studies are needed. Figure 7.2 outlines a suggested approach to investigation and interpretation of results. Moreover, a normal full blood count does not exclude ID given that total body iron stores may be depleted before the onset of overt anaemia.

Iron Studies

The primary marker of ID is ferritin and should be the first-line investigation to exclude or confirm ID. It is advisable to measure ferritin in patients presenting with symptoms of ID even in the absence of an identified anaemia to exclude a non-anaemic ID.

There is debate about the exact cut-off for ferritin in excluding ID, but a threshold cut-off below 50 μg/L may provide the best balance between sensitivity and specificity. A higher threshold, up to 100 μg/L, may be appropriate in the presence of inflammatory disease. Ferritin can be difficult to interpret in the context of inflammation (often evidenced by a raised C-reactive protein [CRP]), and therefore a normal or raised ferritin does not necessarily exclude ID. In these cases, the use of transferrin saturation may be helpful in confirming or excluding an ID at a cut-off of <20% (Figure 7.2).

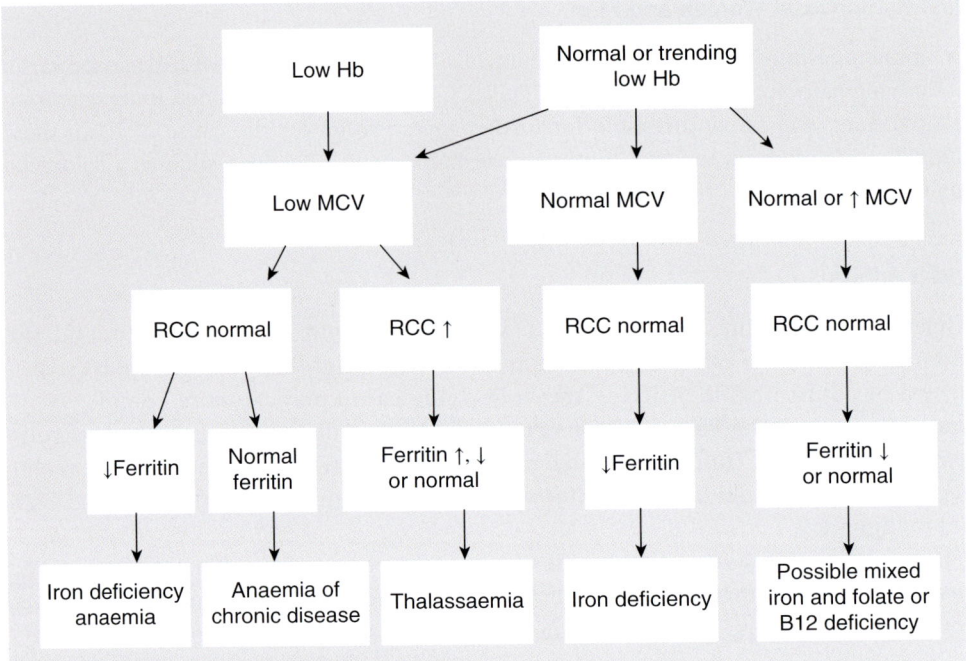

Figure 7.2 Approach to diagnosis of iron deficiency in primary care. RCC, red cell count; Hb, haemoglobin; MCV, mean cell volume.

Further Investigations

In all cases of ID, it is important to test for coeliac disease with tissue transglutaminase (tTG) IgA antibody and endomysial IgA antibody. Antibodies have a high sensitivity particularly in younger individuals.

In pre-menopausal women without any additional symptoms and a history of regular menstrual blood loss, no further investigations are usually required.

In men and post-menopausal women, a full history, medication review and further investigations are usually required to identify an underlying cause. A urine dipstick test is a simple screening test in primary care of occult blood loss from the renal tract that should be undertaken, recognising that sensitivity may be limited.

In approximately 10% of patients with ID anaemia, cancer is found. Therefore, current UK guidance recommends that any adult with ID anaemia is offered faecal immunochemical testing (FIT) to screen for colorectal cancer. If positive, these individuals should be referred urgently for colonoscopy. Those with a negative FIT should also be referred for both gastroscopy and colonoscopy although the urgency of referral will depend on the absolute haemoglobin level.

Treatment of Iron Deficiency in Primary Care

Oral iron should be the first-line treatment option for ID. It is recommended that a daily iron dose of between 40 and 80 mg of elemental iron is needed that, for example, equates to 210 mg of a formulation such as ferrous fumarate (see Chapter 6). This should be continued for approximately 3 months after haemoglobin (if abnormal) has normalised to replenish iron stores.

Side effects are common, and oral iron is often not well tolerated. The dosing of iron can be reduced to once on alternate days, and this may improve gastrointestinal tolerance.

If oral iron is ineffective or not tolerated at all, then intravenous iron is safe and effective and should be considered. A referral to secondary care would normally be needed to instigate intravenous iron.

Dietary Advice and Prevention of Future Iron Deficiency

Whilst increasing dietary iron intake is never sufficient to treat established ID, where ID has been identified and treated, it is important to advise on maintaining a healthy iron intake to prevent recurrent ID. The richest sources of haem iron in the diet include lean red and white meat and seafood. Dietary sources of non-haem iron include nuts, seeds, beans, vegetables and fortified grain products such as bread and cereals. The iron in breast milk is highly bioavailable, but quantities become insufficient to meet the needs of infants older than 4–6 months.

It is also advisable to consume foods rich in vitamin C (such as citrus fruits and green vegetables) to enhance iron absorption. Cooking in cast-iron cookware can increase the iron content of a meal.

Conversely, identifying any substances that might reduce the absorption of iron is important. Common foods and drinks that may do this are tea (containing tannins), coffee and phytate or calcium-rich foods. Levothyroxine, which is commonly prescribed in primary care, can also reduce iron absorption.

Bibliography

Monahan, K.J., Davies, M.M., Abulafi, M. et al. (2022). Faecal immunochemical testing (FIT) in patients with signs or symptoms of suspected colorectal cancer (CRC): a joint guideline from the Association of Coloproctology of Great Britain and Ireland (ACPGBI) and the British Society of Gastroenterology (BSG). *Gut* 71 (10): 1939–1962.

Pratt, J.J. and Khan, K.S. (2016). Non-anaemic iron deficiency–a disease looking for recognition of diagnosis: a systematic review. *European Journal of Haematology* 96 (6): 618–628.

Short, M.W. and Domagalski, J.E. (2013). Iron deficiency anemia: evaluation and management. *American Family Physician* 87 (2): 98–104.

Snook, J., Bhala, N., Beales, I.L. et al. (2021). British Society of Gastroenterology guidelines for the management of iron deficiency anaemia in adults. *Gut* 70 (11): 2030–2051.

The National Institute of Health (NIH), Office of Dietary Supplements (ODS) (2023). Iron – Health Professional Fact Sheet. https://ods.od.nih.gov/factsheets/Iron-Health Professional/

8

Iron Deficiency in the Preoperative Patient

Caroline R. Evans

Department of Anaesthetics, Cardiff and Vale University Healthboard, Cardiff, UK

Introduction

In the preoperative setting, the prevalence of anaemia varies, depending upon the surgical specialty but it is thought to be between 20 and 45%. These patients have worse surgical outcomes than non-anaemic patients, although it is unclear whether this is simply a reflection of the higher disease burden in those with anaemia. Studies investigating the aetiology of anaemia show that ID is the most common cause and lack of available iron, with or without anaemia, is prevalent in up to 80% of patients having major surgical interventions.

Haemoglobin Thresholds

Anaemia is defined as haemoglobin (Hb) of 120 g/L in non-pregnant women and 130 g/L in men. Screening for anaemia prior to surgery is part of the standard workup for an operative procedure. The World Health Organisation (WHO) definition has been challenged in the preoperative setting, suggesting that 120 g/L in women is too low, given that the potential volume of blood loss is the same regardless of sex. By using the WHO definition, women are more likely to reach the transfusion threshold sooner, exposing them to the additive risks of an allogeneic blood transfusion. Countries and health organisations with more established preoperative protocols, and that adopt a patient blood management (PBM) strategy across the surgical pathway, support the definition of anaemia as Hb of 130 g/L in both sexes (Chapter 15). In the United Kingdom, this threshold is included in the guidelines from the British Society of Haematology (BSH) and those from the Centre for Perioperative Care (CPOC), a large multidisciplinary organisation supporting the principle of PBM and a higher Hb threshold for screening.

Iron in Clinical Practice, First Edition. Edited by Sue Pavord and Noemi Roy.
© 2025 John Wiley & Sons Ltd. Published 2025 by John Wiley & Sons Ltd.
Companion website: www.wiley.com/go/medicine5e

Causes of Iron Deficiency in the Surgical Setting

The causes of iron deficiency (ID) in surgical setting are multifactorial and arise from increased loss, such as intestinal or gynaecological bleeding, reduced intake in the diet and/or reduced absorption, and utilisation as seen with functional iron deficiency (FID). FID secondary to inflammation may be related to the presenting surgical condition and other significant patient comorbidities. Upregulation of cytokines in any inflammatory condition, including sepsis, leads to increased production of hepcidin, the hormone that regulates iron trafficking. Understanding the role played by hepcidin (see Chapter 2) is essential to understand the relevant screening tests needed in the surgical setting.

Laboratory Tests

Tests to support the screening for ID help identify the cause and enable appropriate treatment or other diagnostic tests to be organised prior to surgery. Serum ferritin and percent transferrin saturation (TSAT) are simple preoperative screening tests for ID. C-reactive protein and serum creatinine or estimated glomerular filtration rate are required to help characterise the type of ID if serum ferritin is normal. An example of recommended tests and subsequent treatment options is shown in Figure 8.1. Any patient identified as anaemic with a serum ferritin <30 mcg/L, or a serum ferritin of 30–100 mcg/L and TSAT of <20%, should be offered iron

Guideline for the management of Anaemia in the Perioperative Pathway

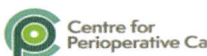

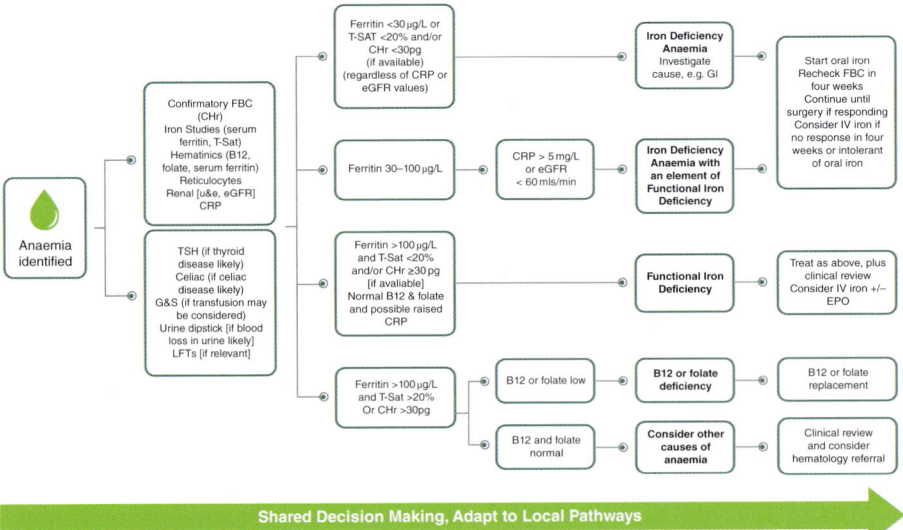

Figure 8.1   Centre for Perioperative Care guideline for the management of anaemia in the perioperative pathway.

treatment prior to major surgery. Recommendations in the National Institute for Health and Care Excellence (NICE) guidelines, NG180 and specifically Quality Standard 138 highlight the need for all surgical patients to be screened for ID and offered iron treatment if needed.

Management of Preoperative Iron Deficiency

Blood transfusion does not appear to ameliorate the risk imposed by anaemia at surgery and may in fact increase postoperative complications and duration of hospital stay. Allogeneic blood transfusion in the preoperative setting should be avoided wherever possible and should be used for major haemorrhage. Indeed, transfusing patients for nutrient deficiency such as ID is reportable to the Serious Hazards of Transfusion (SHOT).

Thus, all current relevant guidelines recommend screening for ID at the point of referral for surgery. The time given to potentially optimise patients differs between surgical specialties and whether patients are on an urgent or elective surgical pathway. However, in many cases, ID is easily modifiable prior to surgery and has led to publication of key guidelines, expert consensus opinion papers and randomised controlled trials investigating the outcomes of the treatment of anaemia and ID in the perioperative setting.

Iron Treatment

Whether oral or intravenous iron is required varies dependent on the cause of the ID, presence of anaemia and the timeline for surgical intervention. For patients who present within 6 weeks of surgery and are diagnosed with anaemia and ID, it is recommended that intravenous iron is used to optimise Hb within the short timeframe. A recent meta-analysis supports this approach in all preoperative colorectal cancer patients, showing a reduction in blood transfusion. Further clinical trials are needed to demonstrate the benefits of intravenous iron in other surgical settings although preliminary data show a reduction in readmission rates and recovery of Hb at 8 weeks. Data in the cardiac surgical setting suggest iron treatment may not only be beneficial in terms of reducing transfusion but also have added long-term benefit in patients with heart failure (see Chapter 11).

Oral iron may be an acceptable and cost-effective treatment in patients who have more than 6 weeks of wait for surgery. However, oral iron does not completely replace iron stores or provide sufficient substrate to cover erythropoiesis after major surgical blood loss. These patients require further testing to ascertain the effect of oral iron and may require further visits to hospital, which is a challenge for patients and healthcare systems. Furthermore, patients report unpleasant side effects with oral iron or take other medicines that inhibit the uptake of iron in the gastrointestinal tract making oral iron an ineffective treatment.

Patients identified with FID or inability to transport iron effectively require more thought. Some may have a reasonable response to intravenous iron, or this response may be blunted due to lack of other cofactors needed for red blood cell production, including erythropoietin, B12 and folate. Both CPOC and BSH recommend concomitant substitution of other nutrients if levels are low. In some patients, it is appropriate to use preoperative erythropoietin in those with FID. In these cases, it should be given with intravenous iron supplementation. There is a lack of trial data in this setting, but current guidelines suggest this combined treatment to ensure a target Hb range of 100–120 g/L for those who decline blood transfusion or have red cell antibodies that make it difficult to source compatible blood. This should be undertaken in consultation with haematologists.

Postoperative Management

To cover all aspects of the patient journey, postoperative anaemia should also be considered. Based on the WHO criteria, 90% of patients following major surgery have anaemia. This is most often reflective of perioperative blood loss, but other aetiologies may play a part. Measures to minimise perioperative blood loss are paramount (see Chapter 15). These include stopping or bridging anticoagulants and antiplatelet therapy, use of antifibrinolytics such as tranexamic acid, surgical glues and sealants and use of point-of-care viscoelastic testing where appropriate. Restrictive transfusion policies are preferred once bleeding has been controlled, and patients may benefit from postoperative iron infusion.

Conclusion

In summary, it is recommended that measures should be taken to optimise patients' Hb prior to major surgery, addressing the first pillar of PBM. Screening for anaemia and ID fits within this aim, and all patients for major surgery should be screened at the earliest point in their patient journey, such as in general practice when the initial surgical referral is made. There is clear evidence that iron therapy in some patient groups is beneficial, but further clinical trials are ongoing across surgical specialties. These will be essential to improve our knowledge and treatment of patients with ID in the perioperative setting.

Bibliography

Centre for Perioperative Care (2022). Anaemia in the perioperative pathway 2022. https://cpoc. org.uk/guidelines-resources-guidelines/anaemia-perioperative-pathway

Clevenger, B. and Richards, T. (2015). Preoperative anaemia. *Anaesthesia* 70 (Suppl. 1): 20–28.

Munoz, M., Acheson, A.G., Auerbach, M. et al. (2017). International consensus statement on the perioperative management of anaemia and iron deficiency. *Anaesthesia* 72: 233–247.

Hands, K., Daru, J., Evans, C. et al. (2024). Identification and management of preoperative anaemia in adults. A British Society of Haematology Guideline update. *Br J Haem* 205 (1): 88–99. https://doi.org/10.1111/ bjh.19440.

Lederhuber, H., Massey, L.H., Abeysiri, S. et al. (2024). Preoperative intravenous iron and the risk of blood transfusion in colorectal cancer surgery: meta- analysis of randomised clinical trials. *Br J Surg* 111 (1): https://doi.org/10.1093/bjs/znad320.

9

Iron Deficiency in Gastroenterology

Mohmmed Tauseef Sharip[1] and Nurulamin M. Noor[1,2]

[1] Department of Gastroenterology, Cambridge University Hospitals NHS Foundation Trust, Cambridge, UK
[2] Department of Medicine, University of Cambridge School of Clinical Medicine, Cambridge, UK

Introduction

Iron deficiency anaemia (IDA) is one of the most common causes of referrals to gastroin-testinal (GI) clinical services. The mechanisms of iron deficiency (ID) include insufficient absorption, inadequate dietary intake and GI bleeding, which can be occult. IDA in some conditions such as inflammatory bowel disease (IBD) may result from a combination of all these factors.

Gastrointestinal Causes of Iron Deficiency

There are several potential GI causes for ID (Table 9.1). In particular, in men and post-menopausal women, IDA can often be the first manifestation of an underlying malignant process, and any new, unexplained presentation of IDA warrants a thorough GI evaluation. In particular, with regard to GI cancer, there is clear evidence that delayed diagnosis will allow disease progression such that patients with more advanced stages of disease have worse outcomes. Indeed outcomes from advanced GI cancers remain amongst the worst for all cancers, with 5-year survival rates for advanced stage IV colorectal cancer remaining at around 10%. In line with this, there has been a large global movement towards earlier detection of dysplasia and malignancy, such that early intervention can allow amelioration of disease and prevention of cancer-related death.

Iron in Clinical Practice, First Edition. Edited by Sue Pavord and Noemi Roy.
© 2025 John Wiley & Sons Ltd. Published 2025 by John Wiley & Sons Ltd.
Companion website: www.wiley.com/go/medicine5e

Table 9.1 Common gastrointestinal causes of iron deficiency.

Dietary factors leading to ID

- Malnutrition or reduced intake of iron (strict vegetarian diet or poverty)
- High intake of phytates and polyphenols
- Tea or milk taken with meals
- Pica syndrome
- Rare: chronic use of proton pump inhibitor (PPI) and H2-histamine receptor blocker

Malabsorption leading to ID

- Coeliac disease
- Inflammatory bowel disease (typically ileal-jejunal disease causing IDA and/or anaemia of chronic disease)
- Duodenal resection/gastric bypass surgery
- *Helicobacter pylori* gastritis
- Small bowel bacterial overgrowth
- Rare: autoimmune gastritis

Loss of iron from GI tract

- Upper gastrointestinal blood loss
  - Malignancy
  - Gastric/duodenal ulcer
  - Variceal bleeding
  - Oesophagitis and erosive gastritis
  - Angiodysplasia and vascular ectasia
  - Dieulafoy's lesions (large tortuous artery)
  - Rare: Meckel diverticula, Cameron lesions, gastric antral vascular ectasia (GAVE) and gastric polyp

- Lower gastrointestinal blood loss
  - Malignancy
  - Diverticulitis/diverticulosis
  - Haemorrhoids, anal fissures and rectal ulcers
  - Angiodysplasia
  - Inflammatory bowel disease
  - Bleeding colonic polyp

Other GI-related causes

- Prolonged non-steroidal anti-inflammatory drug use
- Parasitic infection (e.g. hookworm, tapeworm)
- Rare: Hereditary haemorrhagic telangiectasia, congenital iron deficiency (iron-refractory iron deficiency anaemia) and increased hepcidin (TIMPRSS6 gene mutation) may reduce iron absorption

Assessment of Iron Deficiency in Patients with Gastrointestinal Disease

A detailed and comprehensive history including assessment of dietary intake should be performed for all patients presenting with IDA. Specific questions should be focused on symptoms that might point towards a likely GI cause for IDA including rectal bleeding, weight loss, and altered bowel habit. Of note, a comprehensive history and examination can be helpful to exclude other potential non-GI causes of blood loss such as from the renal tract and heavy menstrual bleeding.

Non-anaemic ID may be difficult to identify using ferritin alone, given that this is an acute-phase reactant protein, which is elevated in the presence of active inflammation. Patients with GI malignancy or IBD often have a functional ID, with iron trapped in entero-cytes, macrophages and hepatocytes due to elevated hepcidin levels. In these clinical set-tings, other blood tests, such as percent transferrin saturation and measurement of soluble transferrin receptors, can be helpful.

Specific Gastrointestinal Investigations

All patients with IDA should be tested for coeliac disease, which is reported to account for 3–5% of all unexplained cases of IDA. Antibodies to tissue transglutaminase (tTG) immu-noglobulin A have high sensitivity and specificity for coeliac disease, with a high negative prediction value (99.6%) – making this a good initial screening test. A definitive test for coeliac disease is duodenal biopsy showing villous atrophy (Figure 9.1).

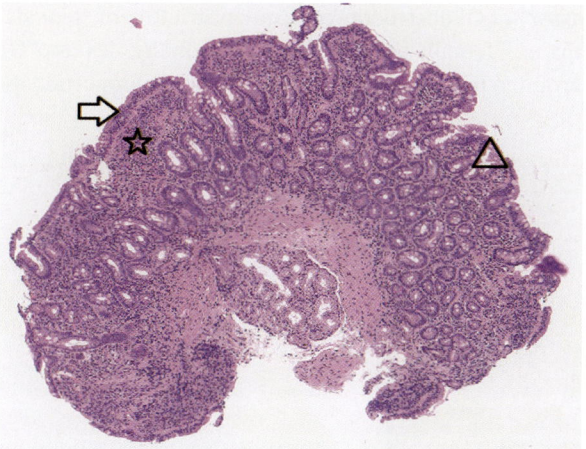

Figure 9.1 Histopathological image showing villous atrophy (triangle), intraepithelial lymphocytosis (arrow) and plasmacytosis (star) in coeliac disease. *Source:* Courtesy of Dr James Chan.

For new-onset IDA in males and postmenopausal women, without any obvious other explainable cause, oesophageal gastroduodenoscopy (OGD) and colonoscopy should be considered. A faecal immunochemical test (FIT) may also be performed to help stratify the urgency of when to perform a colonoscopy. High levels on a quantitative FIT assay would raise the prior probability for a potential GI malignancy. Mildly raised or normal levels on a FIT assay make the likelihood of a GI malignancy less, but do not negate the need for endoscopic assessment, given the possibility of false-negative FIT results.

GI malignancy is only found in 8–10% of cases of IDA, and the majority of endoscopic investigations in such patients do not reveal any significant pathology. Performing an OGD and colonoscopy simultaneously is more convenient than performing them sequentially on different days. There are multiple reasons for this but from a practical point of view, this saves patients the burden of procedures on different days, including preparation for the procedures, and the relatively common instances of dual pathology being found. For those instances where an OGD is initially performed in isolation for IDA, if no abnormality is detected, it should be followed up by a colonoscopy. Figures 9.2–9.5 show upper and lower GI lesions.

For patients who are elderly, frail, and may not tolerate a full colonoscopy procedure, then a reasonable alternative is a CT colonoscopy that is a less-invasive procedure. However, it should be noted that an abnormal CT colonoscopy will typically need to be followed up with a conventional colonoscopy for any biopsies or potential therapeutic endoscopic intervention.

Most patients do not need further investigations at this stage. However, if a patient remains symptomatic despite a trial of iron supplementation or if symptoms recur, further evaluation of the small bowel would be warranted. In this regard, video capsule endoscopy (VCE) is the preferred test for investigating the small bowel as it is highly sensitive to detecting mucosal lesions. Alternatives to VCE include cross-sectional imaging with CT or MRI scans. Cross-sectional imaging is particularly helpful in patients where VCE may not be suitable, such as for those with a history of GI obstruction or known stricture or stenosis.

Although less common, premenopausal female patients can occasionally develop GI malignancy, and GI investigation is warranted in cases where the anaemia is disproportionate

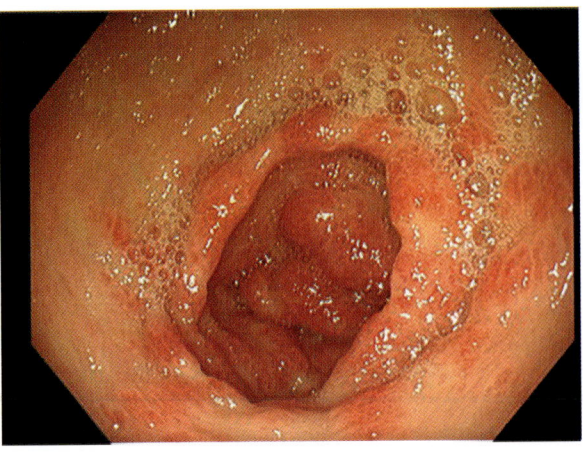

Figure 9.2 Endoscopic image of gastric antral vascular ectasia (GAVE). *Source:* Courtesy of Dr Mohmmed Tauseef Sharip.

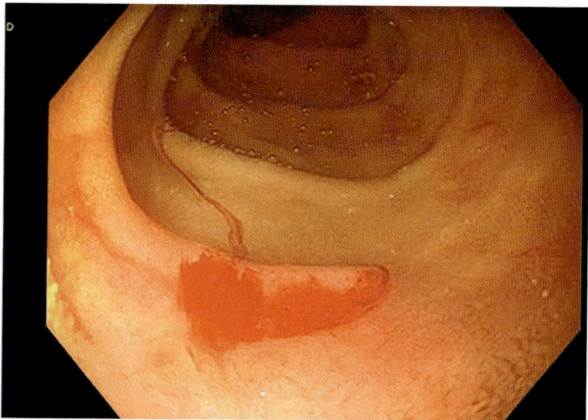

Figure 9.3 Endoscopic image of a bleeding duodenal Dieulafoy's lesion. *Source:* Courtesy of Dr Gareth Corbett.

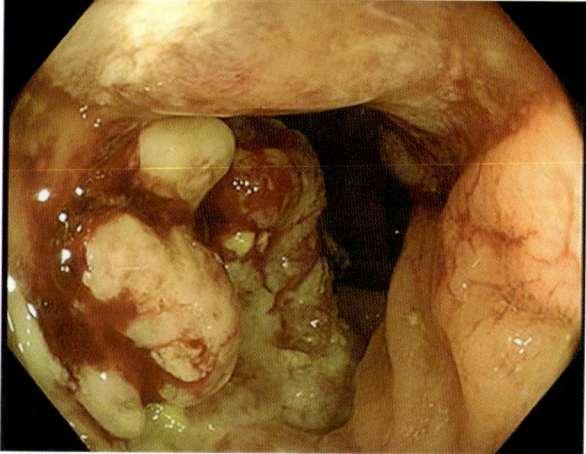

Figure 9.4 Endoscopic image of an ascending colon malignancy. *Source:* Courtesy of Dr De La Revilla Negro.

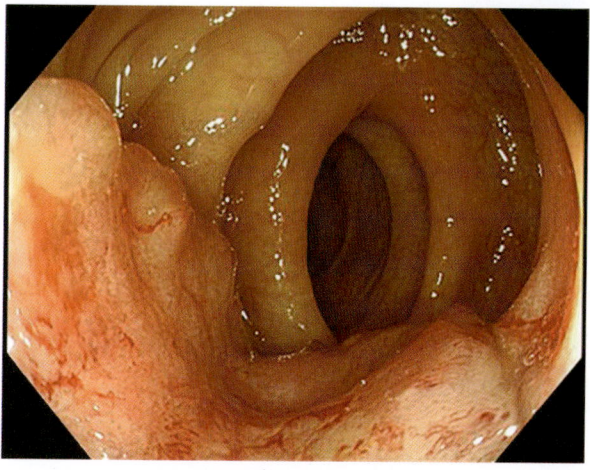

Figure 9.5 Endoscopic image of rectal cancer. *Source:* Courtesy of Dr De La Revilla Negro.

to reported menstrual losses. The presence of any red flag features such as weight loss, change of bowel habit, abdominal mass or a family history of early GI cancer (before the age of 50) should be routinely investigated with both an OGD and colonoscopy. For patients with early-onset colorectal cancer, assessment for DNA mismatch repair gene mutations should be considered to look for any contributing hereditary colorectal cancer syndrome.

Angiodysplasia

Angiodysplasia is an important occult cause of IDA to be aware of particularly in elderly patients. Angiodysplastic vascular lesions are clusters of dilated submucosal vessels that typically occur in the small bowel (Figure 9.6). Although the exact epidemiology is unknown, they appear to become more common with age, mainly above the age of 60 years. Most angiodysplastic lesions are asymptomatic but may present with bleeding into the GI tract, accounting for approximately 1% of such cases. Given their location in the small bowel, they can remain undetected in the face of normal OGD and colonoscopy procedures. A VCE procedure is often the best test to identify angiodysplastic areas; however, their appearances can be subtle and they may only intermittently bleed, making their detection difficult.

Treatment of Iron Deficiency in Patients with Gastrointestinal Disease

Treatment for ID in GI conditions is iron replacement therapy. Unless investigations such as colonoscopy are due to take place imminently, iron replacement therapy should be started immediately whilst patients are awaiting further investigations.

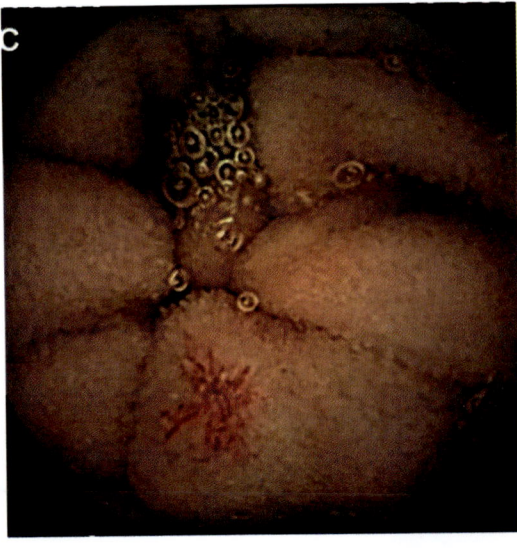

Figure 9.6 Video capsule endoscopic image of small bowel angiodysplasia. *Source:* Courtesy of Dr Gareth Corbett.

Oral iron supplementation is effective in patients with a low serum ferritin, who have an absolute ID from GI blood loss. A satisfactory rise in haemoglobin is typically expected within 2 weeks of starting iron replacement therapy unless there is an ongoing cause of GI bleed or disease. Absorption is low if taken with food, which can reduce bioavailability by up to 75%. Oral iron should be stopped at least one week prior to colonoscopy, to avoid impairing views of the bowel wall and mucosal surface.

Oral iron has reduced efficacy in patients with functional ID, where ferritin levels are normal or high, as elevated hepcidin degrades ferroportin and the absorbed iron is trapped inside the intestinal cell unavailable for use (see Chapter 2). These patients need iron to be given intravenously. Intravenous iron should also be considered for patients who are unable to tolerate oral iron, have recurrent or refractory IDA or need more rapid correction. It is also helpful where oral iron may worsen symptoms, such as for patients with flares of IBD.

All patients starting iron replacement therapy should have haemoglobin checked ideally after 2–4 weeks. Once the haemoglobin reaches the target level, iron replacement should continue for a further 3–6 months to replenish bone marrow stores of iron. Thereafter, patients should have periodic monitoring of their haemoglobin and iron profile, to detect recurrent ID. Figure 9.7 shows a pathway for investigating and managing ID in GI disease.

Blood transfusion should not be used for anaemia due to ID, unless there is concurrent angina, heart failure or cerebral hypoxia. In such cases, one unit of red cells is usually sufficient and can be given on the same day as an iron infusion. After a unit of blood, a clinical and laboratory review is needed to determine the need for another unit. More than one unit should never be given routinely without review. Occasionally, patients with recurrent IDA may need long-term oral iron replacement or periodic IV iron infusions.

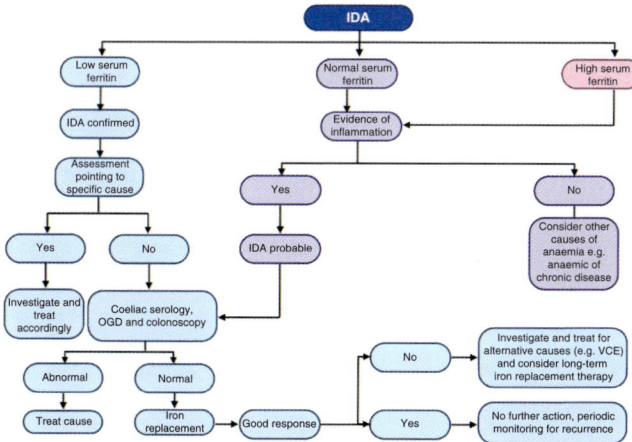

Figure 9.7 Flowchart for the investigation and management of IDA in gastroenterology. VCE, video capsule endoscopy.

Bibliography

DeLoughery, T.G., Jackson, C.S., Ko, C.W., and Rockey, D.C. (2024). AGA Clinical Practice Update on Management of Iron Deficiency Anemia: Expert Review. *Clin Gastroenterol Hepatol* https://doi.org/10.1016/j.cgh.2024.03.046.

GBD (2019). Colorectal cancer collaborators. Global, regional, and national burden of colorectal cancer and its risk factors, 1990–2019: a systematic analysis for the Global Burden of Disease Study 2019. *Lancet Gastroenterol Hepatol* 7 (7): 627–647 (2022).

Gordon, H., Burisch, J., Ellul, P. et al. (2024). ECCO guidelines on extraintestinal manifestations in inflammatory bowel disease. *J Crohns Colitis* 18 (1): 1–37.

Monahan, K.J., Bradshaw, N., Dolwani, S. et al. (2020). Guidelines for the management of hereditary colorectal cancer from the British Society of Gastroenterology (BSG)/Association of Coloproctology of Great Britain and Ireland (ACPGBI)/United Kingdom Cancer Genetics Group (UKCGG). *Gut* 69 (3): 411–444.

Monahan, K.J., Davies, M.M., Abulafi, M. et al. (2022). Faecal immunochemical testing (FIT) in patients with signs or symptoms of suspected colorectal cancer (CRC): a joint guideline from the Association of Coloproctology of Great Britain and Ireland (ACPGBI) and the British Society of Gastroenterology (BSG). *Gut* 71 (10): 1939–1962.

Snook, J., Bhala, N., Beales, I.L.P. et al. (2021). British Society of Gastroenterology guidelines for the management of iron deficiency anaemia in adults. *Gut* 70 (11): 2030–2051.

10

Iron Deficiency in Renal Medicine

Philip A. Kalra

Department of Nephrology, Salford Royal Hospital, Northern Care Alliance NHS Foundation Trust, UK

Introduction

Kidney patients are a group in whom iron deficiency is frequently seen, and use of intravenous (IV) iron is routine in nephrology. However, there are several patient subgroups within nephrology, and iron requirements, targets and treatment regimes differ. This is especially so between those undergoing haemodialysis treatment and patients either treated with peritoneal dialysis (PD) or having their non-dialysis-dependent chronic kidney disease (NDD-CKD) managed. Even the latter sub-group can be divided into those with early- or late-stage NDD-CKD, and iron management can differ in these categories.

Types of Iron Used in Nephrology and Safety Considerations

IV iron has been used routinely for over three decades in nephrology to manage iron deficiency anaemia (IDA). In the United Kingdom and Europe, the preparations most frequently used are iron sucrose (IS), ferric derisomaltose (FDI), and ferric carboxymaltose (FCM). Oral irons are prescribed by some nephrologists for CKD patients with relatively well-preserved kidney function.

The current IV iron preparations are all considered to be very safe, with a low risk of serious adverse reactions (see Chapter 6). One specific adverse reaction, more likely to be seen in other specialties, such as gynaecology and gastroenterology, is hypophosphataemia, but it will be mentioned here because its pathophysiology involves the kidneys. FCM is the IV iron preparation most often associated with this condition, and it is believed that increased levels of intact fibroblast growth factor 23 (FGF23) are responsible. FGF23 is a phosphaturic hormone made in osteocytes that inhibits phosphate reabsorption in the renal proximal tubule – this action is dependent on an obligate co-receptor, klotho. In advancing CKD, FGF23 maintains normal plasma phosphate concentrations until advanced stage 4 or stage 5 disease. However, its stimulation by FCM in people with well-preserved kidney function can

Iron in Clinical Practice, First Edition. Edited by Sue Pavord and Noemi Roy.
© 2025 John Wiley & Sons Ltd. Published 2025 by John Wiley & Sons Ltd.
Companion website: www.wiley.com/go/medicine5e

Hypophosphatemia and bone disorder syndrome

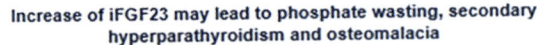

Increase of iFGF23 may lead to phosphate wasting, secondary hyperparathyroidism and osteomalacia

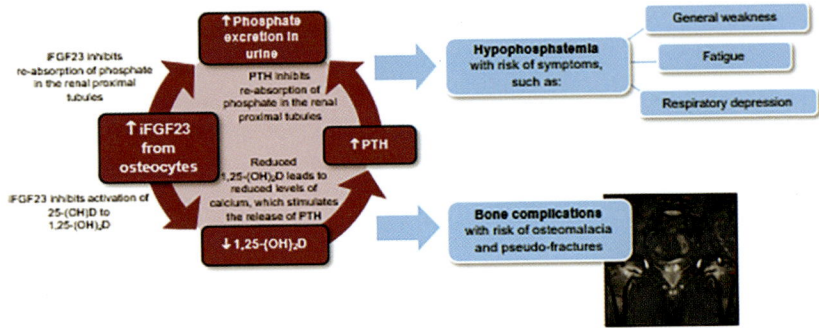

1,25-(OH)2D=1,25-dihydroxyvitamin D; 25-(OH)D=25-hydroxyvitamin D;
iFGF23=intact fibroblast growth factor 23; IV=intravenous; PTH=parathyroid hormone
Adapted from: Expert Opin Drug Saf . 2021 Jul;20(7):757-769

Figure 10.1 Hypophosphatemia and bone disorder syndrome. Increased FGF23 causes downregulation of the 1α-hydroxylase enzyme leading to vitamin D deficiency; cases of osteomalacia have been seen in patients receiving repeated doses of ferric carboxymaltose. X ray *Source:* Heinz Zoller.

often lead to phosphate concentrations <0.6 mmol/L as shown in the PHOSPHARE trial, which compared FCM with FDI in 245 non-CKD patients with IDA. Another effect of FGF23 is downregulation of the 1α-hydroxylase enzyme leading to vitamin D deficiency; cases of osteomalacia have been seen in patients receiving repeated doses of FCM (Figure 10.1).

Longer-term safety concerns with IV iron have included infection risk, based upon the dependence of many pathogens on iron for optimal function, as well as observations that lymphocytes and neutrophils function less well when bathed in high iron concentrations in the laboratory. There is also a hypothetical risk of atherosclerotic cardiovascular disease, based upon the knowledge that the switch between ferric and ferrous iron, due to its redox tendency, can lead to the generation of oxygen-free radicals. However, large randomised controlled trials (RCT) such as PIVOTAL (see next) have provided safety evidence to alleviate these concerns.

Iron Use in Haemodialysis Patients

Soon after the advent of erythropoiesis stimulating agent (ESA) use to address the anaemia suffered by most dialysis patients, it became clear that maintenance of haemoglobin response to ESA was dependent upon regular IV iron treatment. Standard practice subsequently involved bolus injections of IS, given towards the end of a haemodialysis session and into the extracorporeal blood circuit, every 2–4 weeks, depending on iron parameters and haemoglobin response. In the United Kingdom, target ferritin became established at around 400–500 μg/L, with TSat > 20% if achievable.

However, the TREatment of severe Atopic eczema Trial (TREAT) study changed the landscape for iron treatment, especially in North America. Ironically, this was a study testing different ESA regimes and in diabetic NDD-CKD, targeting higher haemoglobin and paying little attention to iron. The primary outcome of the study (mortality and major adverse cardiovascular events (MACE)) was neutral, but secondary outcomes showed a signal of stroke and recurrent cancer in the higher ESA dose arm. Practice in the United States changed, with anaemia care bundles targeting higher ferritin, of around 900–1000 µg/L, to spare ESA doses and hence reduce cardiovascular risk. The PIVOTAL study from the United Kingdom examined the safety of similar high-dose iron regimes, targeting ferritin of up to 700 µg/L versus 200 µg/L in the reactive arm with IS. The result was positive with reduced mortality and MACE in the proactive high-dose arm (Figure 10.2) and reassuringly for safety concerns of IV iron, a significant reduction in myocardial infarction and heart failure hospitalisations with no increase in infection risk. As most haemodialysis patients receive ESA, target haemoglobin is 100–120 g/L as recommended by the European Medicines Agency (EMA).

One frequently encountered issue in dialysis patients in particular is that of functional iron deficiency in which patients have well-preserved or high ferritin but TSat < 20%. These patients typically have ESA unresponsiveness, with requirement for high doses of ESA and sub-optimal haemoglobin response. The mechanism is believed to be hepcidin driven, with this cytokine blocking the iron transport channel in ferroportin and 'locking' iron in macrophages and hepatocytes (Figure 10.3). It is recognised that such patients are at higher all-cause mortality risk. The DRIVE study demonstrated that haemoglobin could be increased in these patients with further high-dose IV iron therapy, targeting ferritin of >1000 µg/L. The newer hypoxia-inducible factor prolyl hydroxylase inhibitors (HIF-PHI) have potential to improve haematopoietic response in some of these patients as they downregulate hepcidin.

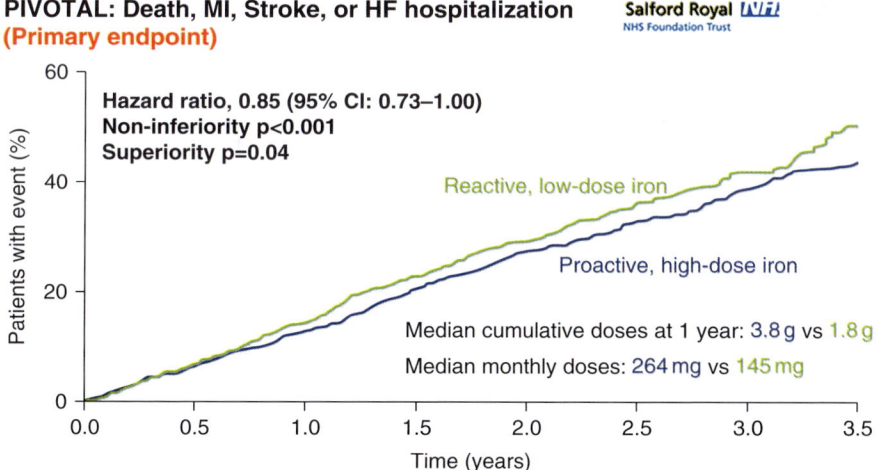

PIVOTAL: Death, MI, Stroke, or HF hospitalization (Primary endpoint)

Hazard ratio, 0.85 (95% CI: 0.73–1.00)
Non-inferiority p<0.001
Superiority p=0.04

Reactive, low-dose iron

Proactive, high-dose iron

Median cumulative doses at 1 year: 3.8 g vs 1.8 g
Median monthly doses: 264 mg vs 145 mg

Hazard ratio (95% CI) adjusted stratification variables: vascular access, diabetic status, and time on dialysis; p value from Wald test.
CI = confidence interval; HF = heart failure; MI = myocardial infarction; PIVOTAL = Proactive IV Iron Therapy in Haemodialysis Patients
Macdougall et al. N Engl J Med. 2019;380(5):447-458. dci: 10.1056\NEJMoa1810742.

Figure 10.2   Results of the PIVOTAL study showing reduced mortality and major adverse cardiovascular events in the haemodialysis cohort treated with high dose intravenous iron. *Source:* Adapted from Macdougall et al. (2019).

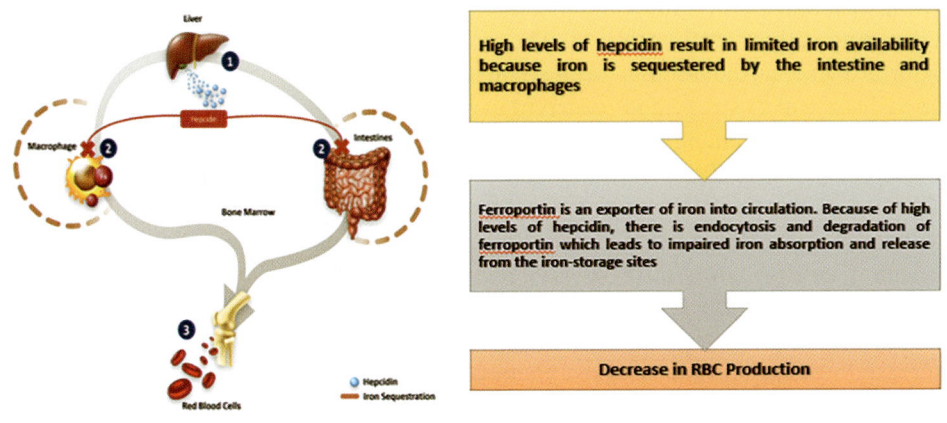

Hepcidin a Key Regulator of Iron

High levels of hepcidin result in limited iron availability because iron is sequestered by the intestine and macrophages

Ferroportin is an exporter of iron into circulation. Because of high levels of hepcidin, there is endocytosis and degradation of ferroportin which leads to impaired iron absorption and release from the iron-storage sites

Decrease in RBC Production

Hain, D., Bednarski, D., Cahill, M., Dix, A., Foote, B., Haras, M.S., Pace, R. and Gutiérrez, O.M., 2023. Iron Deficiency Anemia in CKD: A Narrative Review for the Kidney Care Team. Kidney Medicine, p.100677.

Figure 10.3 High levels of hepcidin produced by the liver, "lock" the iron in the macrophages and intestinal cells. For individuals on dialysis, this may be a reason for resistance to erythropoiesis stimulating agents. *Source:* Hain et al. (2023)/ ELSEVIER /CC-BY-4.0.

Iron Use in Non-Dialysis-Dependent Chronic Kidney Disease

Common definitions of iron deficiency include ferritin <0 mcg/L and TSat <20%. However, for many years, the inflammatory state of CKD, with ferritin recognised to increase as an acute phase response and higher circulating hepcidin, has been used as a lever to choose arbitrary targets of ferritin > 100 μg/L and TSat > 20%. In early CKD, with estimated glomerular filtration rate (eGFR) > 30 mL/min, many patients with IDA can be treated with oral iron with good effect. However, as CKD progresses into stage 4 (eGFR < 30 mL/min), absorption of iron is poorer, and patients are more likely to have gastrointestinal intolerance of oral iron, and hence IV iron is favoured and is preferentially given in single-visit total dose infusions (TDI) such as twould require more than two doses. If the NDD-CKD patient does not require ESA, then there is no upper limit for haemoglobin; ESA-treated patients have a haemoglobin target of ≤120 g/L. Such high-dose regimes have been based on studies such as FIND-CKD with FCM and the PROGRESS study with FDI (Figure 10.4).

Iron Use in Peritoneal Dialysis

The principles of iron treatment in PD patients are broadly similar to those for NDD-CKD patients. Unlike haemodialysis patients who are usually seen by medical practitioners on average three times each week, NDD-CKD and PD patients may only require 3–4 monthly clinic review, and it is important to avoid repeated visits to hospital for patient convenience and avoidance of cross infection. Hence, TDI is recommended for PD patients, and target ferritin is again extrapolated to higher levels, 200–500 μg/L, to reduce ESA need with target haemoglobin again being ≤120 g/L as per EMA guidance.

Change from baseline in Hb concentration over time, by dose (LS mean, 95% CI), FAS

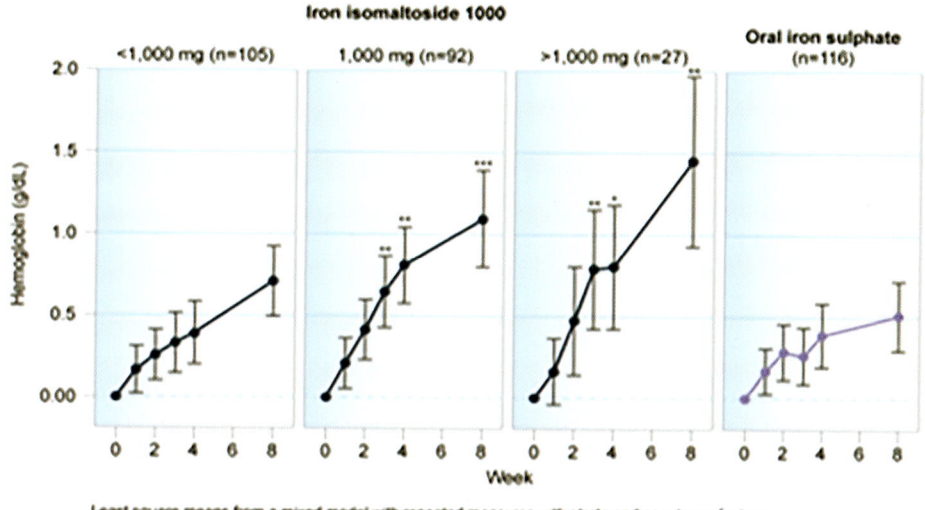

Figure 10.4 A randomised trial of intravenous iron isomaltoside versus oral iron sulphate in patients with non-dialysis-dependent chronic kidney disease with anaemia. Graphs showing the mean change in haemoglobin by dose of intravenous iron isomaltoside or oral iron sulphate. For comparison between iron isomaltoside 1000 mg and oral iron sulphate, p < 0.001. *Source:* Adapted from Kalra et al. (2016).

Bibliography

Hain, D., Bednarski, D., Cavill, M. et al. (2023). Iron deficiency anemia in CKD: a narrative review for the kidney care team. *Kidney Medicine* 100677.

Kalra, P.A., Bhandari, S., Saxena, S. et al. (2016). A randomized trial of iron isomaltoside 1000 versus oral iron in non-dialysis-dependent chronic kidney disease patients with anaemia. *Nephrol Dial Transplant* 31 (4): 646–655.

Macdougall, I.C., Bock, A.H., Carrera, F. et al. (2014). FIND-CKD: a randomized trial of intravenous ferric carboxymaltose versus oral iron in patients with chronic kidney disease and iron deficiency anaemia. *Nephrol Dial Transplant* 29 (11): 2075–2084.

Macdougall, I.C., White, C., Anker, S.D. et al. (2019). Intravenous iron in patients undergoing maintenance hemodialysis. *N Engl J Med* 380 (5): 447–458.

Pfeffer, M.A., Burdmann, E.A., Chen, C.Y. et al. (2009). A trial of darbepoetin alfa in type 2 diabetes and chronic kidney disease. *N Engl J Med* 361 (21): 2019–2032.

Wolf, M., Rubin, J., Achebe, M. et al. (2020). Effects of iron isomaltoside vs ferric carboxymaltose on hypophosphatemia in iron-deficiency anemia: two randomized clinical trials. *JAMA* 323 (5): 432–443.

11

Iron Deficiency in Cardiology

Samira Lakhal-Littleton

Department of Physiology, Anatomy and Genetics, University of Oxford, Oxford, UK

Introduction

Whilst anaemia is a well-established comorbidity in cardiovascular patients, there is growing recognition that iron deficiency (ID) per se, even in the absence of anaemia, can adversely affect these patients. Many prospective studies have revealed that low circulating iron availability predicts increased risk of incident cardiovascular events such as myocardial infarction and stroke and worsens long-term outcomes in those with existing cardiovascular conditions.

Most evidence on the adverse effects of non-anaemic ID has been obtained in the context of heart failure (HF). This chapter will therefore focus on causes, impact and management of ID in HF and will further explore open questions and untapped opportunities in this field.

Both the European Society of Cardiology (ESC) and the American College of Cardiology's (ACC) guidelines now recommend screening HF patients for ID. ESC guidelines define ID as ferritin concentration of either <100 µg/L or <300 µg/L with percentage transferrin saturation (Tsat) < 20%. The rationale for this definition is to encompass both individuals with absolute ID, in whom iron stores are truly depleted (ferritin <100 µg/L) and those with functional ID, in whom inflammation blocks iron absorption from the gut and its mobilisation from stores (ferritin <300 µg/L with Tsat < 20%). Using this definition, the prevalence of ID has been reported at around 75% in acute or decompensated HF, 37–54% in chronic HF (CHF) with reduced ejection fraction (EF) (HFrEF) and 50–64% in CHF with preserved EF (HFpEF).

Causes of Iron Deficiency in Heart Failure

The aetiology of ID in HF is multifactorial. Besides the factors that increase the risk of ID in the general population, i.e. advanced age, female sex, smoking, ethnic background, vegetarian diet and foods rich in phytates and polyphenols, additional factors relevant to HF patients explain the high prevalence of ID in this group. These are summarised in Table 11.1.

Iron in Clinical Practice, First Edition. Edited by Sue Pavord and Noemi Roy.
© 2025 John Wiley & Sons Ltd. Published 2025 by John Wiley & Sons Ltd.
Companion website: www.wiley.com/go/medicine5e

Table 11.1 Causes underpinning high prevalence of ID in HF patients.

Cause	Mechanism
Malnutrition, e.g. due to nausea, swallowing disturbances, or loss of appetite due to fatigue and worsening HF	Low dietary iron intake
Adverse intestinal, mucosal, and bacteria remodelling due to hypoperfusion in patients with venous congestion	Inefficient dietary iron absorption
Long-term use of proton pump inhibitors and histamine-2 receptor antagonists that impair gastric acid production (acid is needed to maintain iron in ferrous form necessary for uptake)	Low bioavailability of dietary iron
Elevation of hepcidin, e.g. inflammatory comorbidities where IL-6 is elevated; chronic kidney disease where plasma hepcidin renal clearance is impaired	Inefficient dietary iron absorption and trapping of iron within stores
Gastrointestinal conditions, e.g. colonic polyps, esophagitis, gastritis, peptic ulcer, or inflammatory bowel disease	Excessive iron loss through gastrointestinal bleeding
Antiplatelets, e.g. aspirin, and anticoagulants, e.g. warfarin	Excessive iron loss through gastrointestinal bleeding
Calcium channel blockers, e.g. amlodipine Sodium-glucose transporter SGLT2 inhibitors, e.g. dapagliflozin	Unknown mechanism

Impact of Iron Deficiency in Heart Failure

In CHF, with either preserved or reduced EF, ID, as defined by ESC guidelines, is associated with reduced exercise capacity, manifesting as a reduction in the distance covered in a 6-minute walk test or in maximal oxygen consumption (VO_2 max). It is also associated with increased risk of recurrent HF hospitalisation, cardiovascular death and all-cause mortality. In patients discharged for acute HF, ferritin $<100\,\mu g/L$ is associated with increased risk of 30-day hospital readmission. In patients with decompensated HF, being in the lowest quartile of TSat% is associated with increased risk of 30-day death or decompensated HF readmission.

Adverse effects of ID are seen even in the absence of anaemia, the hypothesis being that the myocardium becomes iron deficient and that myocardial ID compromises the production of energy needed for heart contraction. Magnetic resonance (MR)-based studies have failed to detect myocardial ID or impaired cardiac energetics in iron-deficient HF patients, though this could reflect the technical limitations of MR-based assessment of tissue iron. On the other hand, biopsy studies suggest that myocardial ID occurs in advanced HF as a result of decreased iron uptake and increased iron export in cardiac myocytes. Preclinical studies provide proof of concept that impaired iron uptake or excessive iron export compromise the contractile function of the heart. Other hypotheses linking ID with HF include skeletal muscle iron depletion resulting in reduced exercise capacity, as well as adverse pulmonary vascular remodelling, resulting in haemodynamic stress on the right heart. These hypotheses are summarised in Figure 11.1.

Management of Iron Deficiency in Heart Failure

Whilst oral iron therapies often improve circulating iron and haematological parameters in HF patients, their effects on functional and clinical outcomes have not been consistent. One potential cause is the relatively low fractional absorption of dietary iron in general

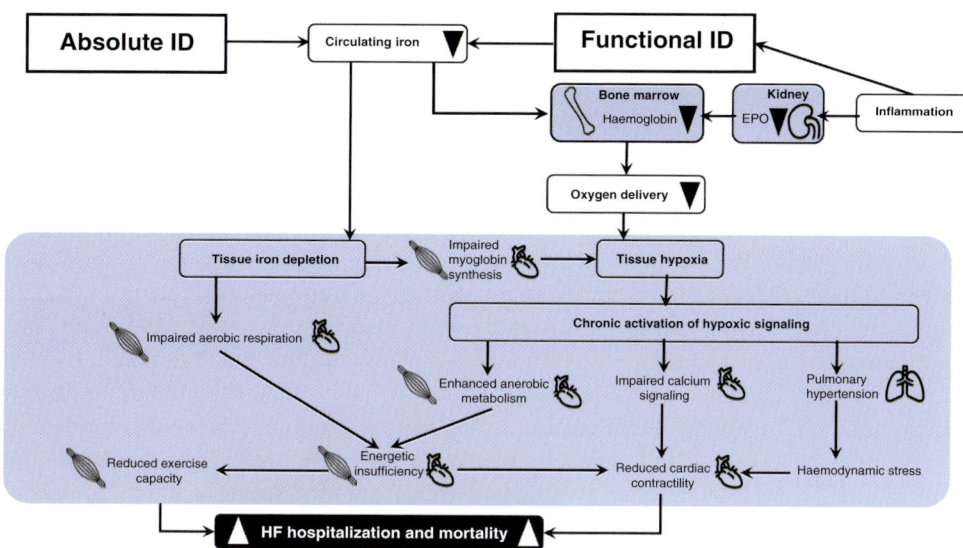

Figure 11.1 Potential mechanisms for the detrimental effect of ID in HF patients.

(in the order of 10–20% from a standard 100 mg dose), which, in inflamed HF patients, may be further compounded by the mucosal block on iron absorption.

Intravenous (IV) iron therapies have produced more consistent benefits in trials, such as reducing the risk of recurrent hospitalisation for HF or cardiovascular death and improving functional capacity, e.g. 6-minute walk test and Max VO_2. Consequently, ESC guidelines now recommend IV iron therapy for symptomatic patients with reduced HFrEF or moderately reduced HFmrEF, that meet its definition of ID. ACC guidelines state that IV iron therapy is 'reasonable' in patients with HFrEF and ID.

The benefits of IV iron therapies in HF patients appear multifactorial. In anaemic patients, IV iron therapy improves exercise capacity, peak VO_2 and sleep-disordered breathing, with the magnitude of improvements relating to the correction of haemoglobin and O_2 delivery to the skeletal muscle. In non-anaemic patients, the mechanisms underlying the benefits of IV iron are not well understood. MR-based studies indicate that these therapies do increase the iron content of the myocardium. However, the contribution of this extra myocardial iron, if any, to improved myocardial function remains unproven.

Diagnostic and Management Uncertainties in Individuals with Cardiac Disease

Current Definitions of Iron Deficiency

There is an ongoing debate as to whether guideline definitions of ID optimally capture HF patients with an unmet need for iron and who derives benefits from iron supplementation. For instance, in anaemic HFrEF patients, Tsat <20% and serum iron ≤13 µmol/L, but not ESC definition, were associated with higher 5-year mortality. The debate about how best to define ID in HF patients reflects, in part, the wider limitations of the clinical iron markers, with both ferritin and TSat% being confounded by inflammation.

Current Iron Replacement Therapies

Knowledge of iron homeostasis has grown exponentially over the past decade, but it is yet to be harnessed for guiding iron replacement therapies. For instance, oral iron therapies in HF patients should be revisited in light of evidence that alternate-day dosing results in greater fractional absorption, as well as the advent of new slow-release formulations, e.g. sucrosomial iron, that appear less sensitive to the mucosal block. The fate of iron from IV iron therapies in inflamed patients warrants further exploration, given that elevated hepcidin would theoretically result in the eventual trapping of iron in stores (Figure 11.2). The safety of repeated IV iron therapy also merits further attention in cardiac patients, in light of evidence that some formulations release iron directly into the circulation and that the myocardium takes up and retains this iron.

In summary, ID is highly prevalent in cardiac patients and associated with a range of adverse outcomes. Tackling it holds immense potential, but unlocking that potential requires better ways of diagnosing true ID and greater understanding of the behaviour of iron replacement therapies in the body.

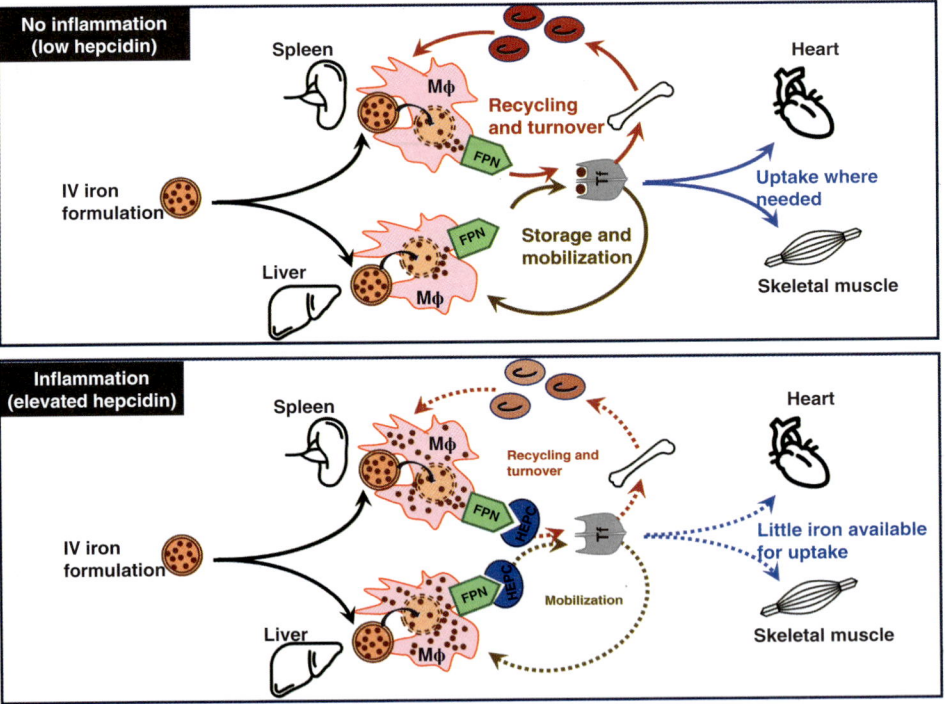

Figure 11.2 Potential impact of inflammation and hepcidin on fate of iron from IV iron therapies. MΦ, macrophage; FPN, ferroportin (iron exporter); Tf, transferrin; HEPC, hepcidin.

Bibliography

Heidenreich PA, Bozkurt B, Aguilar D, Allen LA, Byun JJ, Colvin MM, Deswal A, Drazner MH, Dunlay SM, Evers LR, Fang JC, Fedson SE, Fonarow GC, Hayek SS, Hernandez AF, Khazanie P, Kittleson MM, Lee CS, Link MS, Milano CA, Nnacheta LC, Sandhu AT, Stevenson LW, Vardeny O, Vest AR, Yancy CW. 2022 AHA/ACC/HFSA Guideline for the Management of Heart Failure: A Report of the American College of Cardiology/American Heart Association Joint Committee on Clinical Practice Guidelines. *Circulation.* 2022 May 3;145(18):e895–e1032. doi: https://doi.org/10.1161/CIR.0000000000001063. Erratum in: Circulation. 2022 May 3;145 (18):e1033. Erratum in: Circulation. 2022 Sep 27;146 (13):e185. Erratum in: Circulation. 2023 Apr 4; 147(14): e674.

Lakhal-Littleton, S. and Cleland, J.G.F. (2024). Iron deficiency and supplementation in heart failure. *Nat Rev Cardiol* https://doi.org/10.1038/s41569-024-00988-1.

Lindberg, F., Lund, L.H., Benson, L. et al. (2023). Iron deficiency in heart failure: screening, prevalence, incidence and outcome data from the Swedish Heart Failure Registry and the Stockholm CREAtinine Measurements collaborative project. *Eur J Heart Fail* 25: 1270–1280, https://doi.org/10.1002/ejhf.2879.

Masini, G., Graham, F.J., Pellicori, P. et al. (2022). Criteria for iron deficiency in patients with heart failure. *J Am Coll Cardiol* 79: 341–351, https://doi.org/10.1016/j.jacc.2021.11.039.

McDonagh, T.A., Metra, M., Adamo, M. et al. (2024). 2023 Focused Update of the 2021 ESC Guidelines for the diagnosis and treatment of acute and chronic heart failure: Developed by the task force for the diagnosis and treatment of acute and chronic heart failure of the European Society of Cardiology (ESC) With the special contribution of the Heart Failure Association (HFA) of the ESC. *Eur J Heart Fail* 26 (1): 5–17. https://doi.org/10.1002/ejhf.3024.

Vera-Aviles, M., Kabir, S., Shah, A. et al. Intravenous iron therapy with ferric carboxymaltose results in a rapid and sustained rise in myocardial iron content through a non-canonical pathway: a translational study. *medRxiv* https://doi.org/10.1101/2024.01.18.24301496.

12

Iron Deficiency in Neurology

Carmen Jacob[1,2] and Ian Galea[1,2]

[1] *Clinical Neurosciences, Clinical and Experimental Sciences, Faculty of Medicine, University of Southampton, UK*
[2] *Wessex Neurological Centre, University Hospital Southampton NHS Foundation Trust, UK*

Introduction

Iron plays a crucial role in numerous fundamental processes necessary for normal neurological function, such as mitochondrial respiration, nucleic acid metabolism, redox equilibrium, neurotransmitter synthesis and myelin maturation. Hence, it is not surprising that disruption of brain iron homeostasis causes neurological symptoms. Neurological effects of iron deficiency (ID) may be seen in the absence of anaemia or microcytosis, which suggests that the central nervous system (CNS) may be more sensitive to low iron stores than erythropoiesis. Functional cellular ID, such as with mutations in iron regulatory protein-2 or L-ferritin, results in a neurological phenotype; in the case of L-ferritin, this occurs without haematological abnormalities.

Iron Utilisation in the Central Nervous System

Iron entry into the CNS and its metabolism by neuroglia are tightly regulated (Figure 12.1), as both deficiency and excess of iron impair neurological function. Different cell types in the CNS such as neurons, microglia, astrocytes and oligodendrocytes exchange iron, although details are yet to be understood. Iron is a critical component of metalloproteins involved in energy metabolism, such as respiratory chain complexes in mitochondria. The brain is the topmost energy-consuming organ at rest, mostly due to neuronal activity, accounting for 20% of total body energy and oxygen consumption, despite weighing only 2% of body mass. Given their high energy demands, it is intuitive that neurons may be particularly susceptible to ID. When ID progresses to anaemia, brain tissue becomes more vulnerable to local hypoxia, due to decreased red blood cell oxygen carriage and deformability, accentuating the effects of ID on CNS function. Iron is also essential for iron–sulphur complex-containing enzymes which maintain

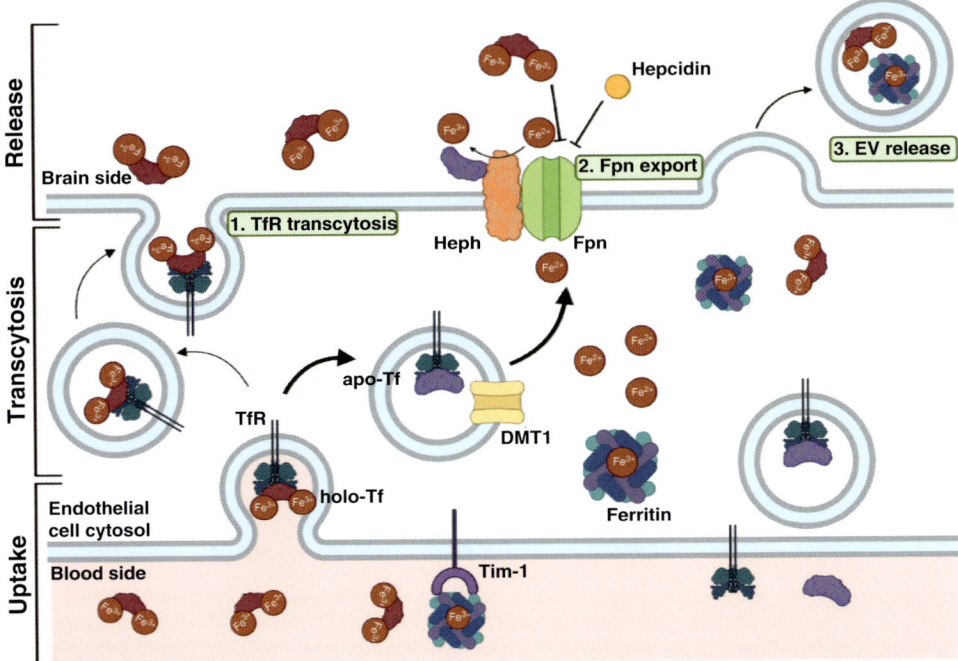

Figure 12.1 Iron uptake in the central nervous system. Iron crosses the endothelial cells (ECs) of the blood–brain barrier (BBB) to enter the CNS whilst bound to transferrin (Tf) in its ferric form, Fe^{3+} (holo-Tf). Iron uptake into ECs is mediated by transferrin receptors (TfR), making TfR availability a key regulatory mechanism for CNS iron homeostasis. Iron may also enter ECs bound to H-ferritin via Tim-1 receptors. Multiple routes into the CNS are then possible. Starting from the left of the diagram, endocytotic vesicles (EVs) containing holo-Tf-TfR complexes can move from the luminal membrane across the EC to fuse with the abluminal membrane and release holo-Tf into the CNS parenchyma (direct transcytosis). A more commonly utilised route is shown in the midline: Fe3+ is released from holo-Tf-TfR complexes due to lowering of intravesical pH, as holo-Tf-TfR complex-containing EVs mature to endosomes, which contain an acidifying ATPase. This is followed by reduction to ferrous iron (Fe^{2+}) by ferrireductases and export from the endosome to the intracellular milieu via divalent metal transporter-1 (DMT1). Free intracellular Fe^{2+} then leaves the EC to enter the CNS via ferroportin (Fpn), immediately after which it is oxidised to Fe^{3+} by hephaestin (Heph) enabling it to bind to Tf within the extracellular milieu of the CNS. In another route, shown on the right, holo-Tf complexes and/or H-ferritin can be bundled as cargo in vesicles budding from the abluminal surface of ECs followed by fusion with astrocytes. *Source:* Baringer et al. (2023)/John Wiley & Sons.

nucleic acid integrity. This is particularly important in neurons since they are long-lived cells with a poor regenerative capacity. Finally, iron is part of a finely balanced redox system and neurons are particularly susceptible to oxidative stress. Amongst all cell types in the CNS, oligodendrocytes have the highest iron concentration, where it is crucial for maturation of oligodendrocyte precursors and synthesis of myelin. Microglia take up extra iron when activated. Both of these processes may act as an iron sink potentially accentuating the effects of ID on neurons during neurodevelopment or pathology.

Iron and Neurocognitive Development

Iron is crucial for ante- and postnatal neurodevelopment. ID impairs a variety of processes, such as neuronal differentiation and proliferation, myelination, synaptic plasticity and dendritic arborisation and is associated with delayed psychomotor development, neurodevelopmental disorders and cognitive impairments. Core structures for learning, such as the hippocampus, are particularly vulnerable to ID. Impairments induced by systemic ID can persist despite normalisation of iron status, and later-onset ID aggravates neurodevelopmental disorders. To prevent the marked effects of ID on ante- and post-natal development, the World Health Organisation recommends iron supplementation in all pregnant women.

Neurological Associations with Iron Deficiency

A number of neurological symptoms or presentations have been reported as having an association with either isolated ID or ID anaemia. Often, it is difficult to ascertain to which extent these symptoms are secondary to anaemia, ID per se, a combination of both, or are the result of a correlation with another factor.

Lethargy and fatigue are the most widely recognised neurological symptoms of ID anaemia. These symptoms are thought to relate in part to ID itself, rather than being solely mediated by anaemia, as iron supplementation in iron-deficient, non-anaemic patients improves fatigue.

Headaches are associated with ID anaemia, hypothesised to be caused by ID-related altered dopaminergic function.

Cognitive impairment (especially with older age) and **psychiatric presentations** such as psychosis, anxiety and affective disorders have been observed with ID. This is possibly explained by iron being a necessary cofactor in the synthesis of monoamines including serotonin, norepinephrine and dopamine. Some studies suggest that iron supplementation may improve general mood, sleep quality, depressive symptoms and cognitive function.

ID is strongly associated with **restless legs syndrome (RLS)**, which in turn is six times more likely with ID anaemia. Even if systemic ID markers are normal, RLS patients may have reduced CNS iron. Whilst mechanisms are incompletely understood, it is thought that CNS ID leads to reduced dopaminergic function causing spinal hyperexcitability and RLS symptoms.

Several large epidemiological studies suggest an increased risk of developing **Parkinson's disease** with anaemia, and a decreased risk with higher serum iron levels, but causality is not established.

ID anaemia has been linked to **cerebral venous sinus thromboses** in paediatric and adult case reports. Patients with **idiopathic intracranial hypertension** (IIH), which can follow cerebral venous sinus thromboses, are almost twice as likely to be anaemic, such that 18% have anaemia, mostly commonly of the ID type. When IIH and anaemia coexist, treatment of anaemia alone will resolve IIH in more than half.

ID anaemia is associated with higher odds of **sensorineural and combined hearing loss** in children and adults. Hypothesised explanations include ischaemic damage and reduced myelin production. **Neurophysiological changes** associated with ID, particularly in children, include prolonged visually evoked potential latencies and reduced peripheral sensory and motor conduction velocities. Normalisation of neurophysiological parameters is reported following iron supplementation in some studies.

Recommendations for Management of Iron Deficiency with Neurological Symptoms

Given the variety of neurological symptoms reported to be associated with ID, clinicians should have a low threshold to investigate iron status. There are no general guidelines for the assessment and management of ID with neurological symptoms. However, specific guidelines exist in RLS. A morning, fasting iron panel including serum iron, ferritin, total iron binding capacity and transferrin saturation is recommended. Importantly, a normal full blood count is insufficient to exclude ID, as neurological symptoms may be seen in non-anaemic ID. Given the postulated higher sensitivity of the nervous system to low iron stores, early iron supplementation in patients with low-normal ferritin levels (i.e. <75µg/L) may be beneficial. To avoid peripheral iron overload in susceptible individuals when supplementing iron without evidence of systemic ID, iron status should be monitored regularly. Iron supplementation should be avoided if transferrin saturation is >45% and/or ferritin is >300µg/L. Investigations should be considered to exclude secondary ID.

Conclusion

ID impairs neurological function in multiple ways and can contribute to a variety of neurological symptoms. Whilst details of the underlying pathophysiological mechanisms remain incompletely understood, clinicians should consider that the neurological system might be more susceptible to ID and have a low threshold to investigate iron status in primary and secondary care, even in non-anaemic patients.

Bibliography

Allen, R.P., Picchietti, D.L., Auerbach, M. et al. (2018). Evidence-based and consensus clinical practice guidelines for the iron treatment of restless legs syndrome/Willis-Ekbom disease in adults and children: an IRLSSG task force report. *Sleep Med* 41: 27–44.

Baringer, S.L., Simpson, I.A., and Connor, J.R. (2023). Brain iron acquisition: an overview of homeostatic regulation and disease dysregulation. *J Neurochem* 165: 625–642.

Levi, S., Ripamonti, M., Moro, A.S., and Cozzi, A. (2024). Iron imbalance in neurodegeneration. *Mol Psychiatry* 29: 1139–1152.

Levin, S. (2023). Iron deficiency in psychiatric patients. *Curr Psychiatr* 22: 29–34.

Mcwilliams, S., Singh, I., Leung, W. et al. (2022). Iron deficiency and common neurodevelopmental disorders-A scoping review. *PLoS One* 17: e0273819.

Pivina, L., Semenova, Y., Doşa, M.D. et al. (2019). Iron deficiency, cognitive functions, and neurobehavioral disorders in children. *J Mol Neurosci* 68: 1–10.

Saadatnia, M., Fatehi, F., Basiri, K. et al. (2009). Cerebral venous sinus thrombosis risk factors. *Int J Stroke* 4: 111–123.

Ward, R.J., Zucca, F.A., Duyn, J.H. et al. (2014). The role of iron in brain ageing and neurodegenerative disorders. *Lancet Neurol* 13: 1045–1060.

Yavuz, B.B., Cankurtaran, M., Haznedaroglu, I.C. et al. (2012). Iron deficiency can cause cognitive impairment in geriatric patients. *J Nutr Health Aging* 16: 220–224.

Yu, C.W., Waisberg, E., Kwok, J.M., and Micieli, J.A. (2022). Anemia and idiopathic intracranial hypertension: a systematic review and meta-analysis. *J Neuroophthalmol* 42: e78–e86.

13

Iron Deficiency in Obstetrics

Sue Pavord

Department of Haematology, Oxford University Hospitals NHS Foundation Trust, Oxford, UK

Introduction

Iron deficiency anaemia is the most common medical disorder seen in the obstetric setting, occurring in over 40% of pregnant women worldwide. Prevalence is highest in low- and middle-income countries, where it can be over 50%, but for every country it is a significant public health issue, even if it has not yet been recognised as such.

Non-pregnant women of child-bearing age are commonly iron deficient due to a combination of regular menstruation and poor dietary intake. In pregnancy, due to the increasing demand for iron (Figure 13.1), the recommended daily intake increases from 8 mg/day to 27 mg/day. For most women this is not achievable, even though absorption capacity increases due to reduced hepcidin levels in the antepartum period (Figure 13.2). So with inadequate reserves and inability to sufficiently increase iron intake, many women become iron depleted in pregnancy if not provided with supplementation.

The Maternal Effects of Iron Deficiency

As iron is needed for normal functioning of every cell in the body, it's not surprising that anaemic women may suffer with fatigue, breathlessness, cognitive and immune dysfunction. In many cases they may have attributed this to the pregnancy itself or caring for young children. Pica and pagophagia are also common and usually resolve rapidly after iron replacement.

More seriously, iron-depleted women are at increased risk of postpartum haemorrhage; the lower the haemoglobin, the greater the estimated blood loss. This is likely due to reduced uterine contractility, but mild coagulation impairment has also been seen in severely iron-deficient women. Large epidemiological studies from the World Health Organisation's database, which adjusted for confounding factors, revealed a twofold increase in mortality when haemoglobin has been below 70 g/L during or after pregnancy.

Iron in Clinical Practice, First Edition. Edited by Sue Pavord and Noemi Roy.
© 2025 John Wiley & Sons Ltd. Published 2025 by John Wiley & Sons Ltd.
Companion website: www.wiley.com/go/medicine5e

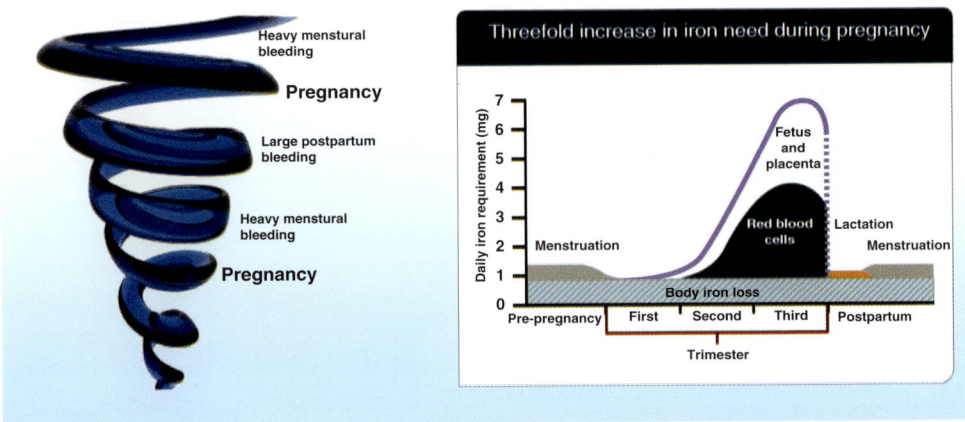

Figure 13.1 Iron requirements in pregnancy and the negative iron spiral in fertile life.
Source: Adapted from Bothwell (2000) and Milman et al. (2017).

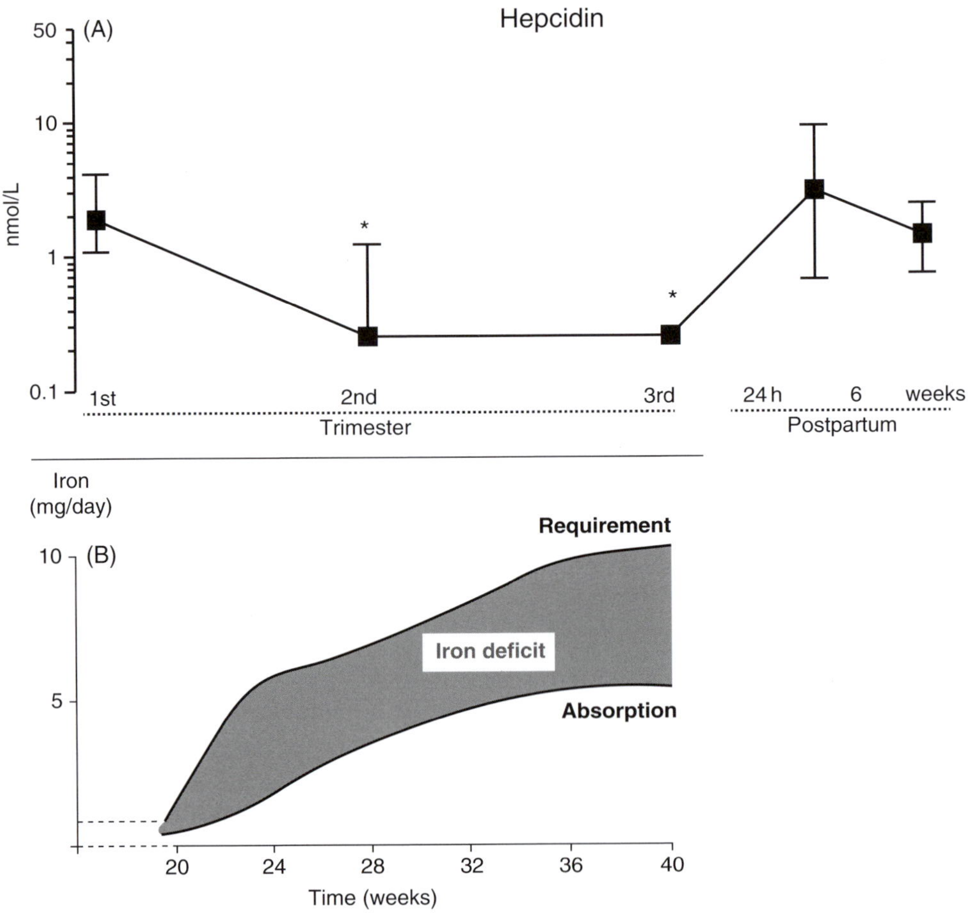

Figure 13.2 A. Maternal hepcidin concentrations are decreased in the second and third trimesters, allowing an increased supply of iron to the fetus. * p<0.0001 compared to first trimester values. *Source:* van Santen et al. (2013). B. The increased demand for iron is greater than the increased capacity for absorption, causing an iron deficit to expand. *Source:* World Health Organisation and Food and Agriculture Organisation of the United Nations (2002).

In the postpartum period, fatigue, depression and mother–child interactions have been shown to improve with iron supplementation.

Fetal Effects of Iron Deficiency

Maternal-to-fetal transfer of iron is largely in the last 4–5 weeks of gestation. Despite the preferential delivery of iron to the fetus, a point is reached when the fetus may also be compromised and low cord ferritin levels have been noted when maternal serum ferritin is below 13 mcg/L. Importantly for the fetus, is the iron requirement for brain development, neurotransmitter synthesis and myelin production, and observational studies have found lower Apgar scores and poor cognition in babies born to iron-deficient mothers. Maternal anaemia has also been associated with low birth weight and prematurity.

Defining Anaemia in Pregnancy

Blood volume increases by around 1.5 L in pregnancy, to meet the demands of the placental vascular bed. A physiological haemodilution occurs due to a disproportionate expansion of the plasma volume relative to expansion of the red cell mass – the former being twice that of the latter. This haemodilutional change is not linear as pregnancy advances but rather has an S-shaped curve, beginning at the start of the second trimester and reaching a peak at end of it (Figure 13.3). Consequently, the definitions of anaemia are revised downwards and anaemia is considered to be present when Hb is lower than 110 g/L in the antenatal period and less than 100 g/L in the immediate postpartum period, although these definitions are under review.

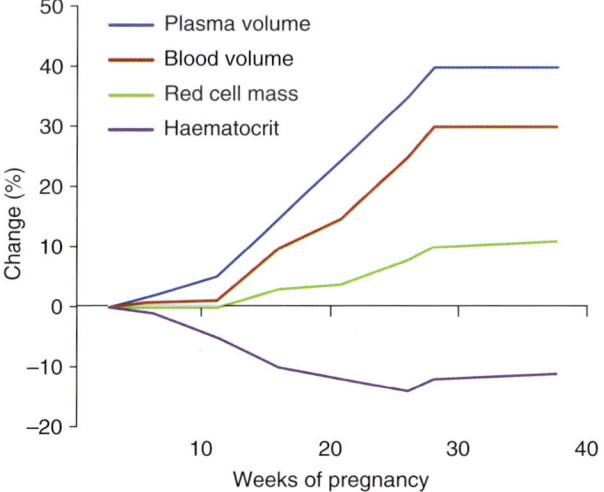

Figure 13.3 Blood volume changes in pregnancy.

Table 13.1 Risk factors for iron deficiency in pregnancy.

Previous anaemia

Interpregnancy interval <1 year

Twin or higher-order multiple pregnancy

Multiparity ≥3

Recent history of clinically significant bleeding

Women with a high intake of tea, dairy, cereals and chapati along with main meal

Those following a vegetarian/vegan diet

Pregnant teenagers

How Is Iron Deficiency Diagnosed in Pregnancy?

Standard tests of iron status each have limitations in pregnancy. Serum ferritin may be considered as the current gold standard, but whilst a low serum ferritin is diagnostic of iron deficiency, a normal level does not exclude it. Ferritin is elevated by underlying inflammation, infection, recent iron ingestion and may be altered in normal pregnancy itself. Red cell indices are not helpful and mean cell volume rises by around 6fl in normal pregnancy. Other biomarkers of iron status have not been validated. Guidance from the British Society for Haematology is to use a trial of oral iron as a diagnostic tool, assessing improvement in Hb after 2–4 weeks. Non-anaemic iron deficiency is common, and risk factors should be considered, with a low threshold applied for administration of oral iron (Table 13.1). Ferritin should be checked in women with known haemoglobinopathy to exclude an iron-loading state.

Indications for Intravenous Iron

Intravenous (IV) iron has the advantage of rapid repletion of iron status, avoidance of gastrointestinal side effects and confirming compliance. The lipid-bound preparations can be given as 1g or more (depending on the preparation) over 15 minutes, with <1 : 10,000 risk of anaphylaxis. IV iron should not be given in the first trimester due to potential toxicity to trophoblastic tissue. It is beneficial for those presenting after 34 weeks' gestation with Hb <100 g/L where there is insufficient remaining time before delivery for correction of anaemia with oral iron and similarly for those with profound iron deficiency (such as ferritin <10 mcg/L) at any gestation. After iron infusion, oral iron should be resumed around two weeks later, when hepcidin levels have declined to baseline and absorption is no longer impaired. Absorption, and therefore tolerance, can be significantly improved by correct administration, no more than one tablet every morning, taken with water or orange juice on an empty stomach an hour before food, drink, multivitamins and other medications.

Management of Postpartum Anaemia

Women at risk of postpartum anaemia because of blood loss of >500 mL, uncorrected antenatal anaemia or symptoms consistent with anaemia should have their Hb checked within 48 hours of delivery. If anaemia is confirmed, iron replacement with oral or IV iron should be initiated. Blood transfusion should be avoided unless there is cardiovascular compromise or significant risk of rebleeding and Hb is <70 g/L. Transfusion carries appreciable risks of adverse events including red cell alloimmunisation with future risk of haemolytic disease of the fetus/newborn, as well as potential difficulty obtaining compatible blood.

Bibliography

American College of Obstetricians and Gynecologists (2021). Anemia in pregnancy: ACOG practice bulletin, number 233. *Obstet Gynecol* 138 (2): e55–e64.

Bothwell, T.H. (2000). Iron requirements in pregnancy and strategies to meet them. *Am J Clin Nutr* 72 (suppl): 257S–264S.

Daru, J., Zamora, J., Fernandez-Felix, B.M. et al. (2018). Risk of maternal mortality in women with severe anaemia during pregnancy and post partum: a multilevel analysis. *Lancet Glob Health* 6: e548–e554.

Georgieff, M.K. (2020). Iron deficiency in pregnancy. *Am J Obstet Gynecol* 223 (4): 516–524.

Green, L., Connolly, C., Cooper, T.K., et al. (2015). Blood transfusion in obstetrics. Royal College of Obstericians and Gynaecologists Greentop guideline no 47.

Milman, N., Taylor, C.L., Merkel, J., and Brannon, P.M. (2017). Iron status in pregnant women and women of reproductive age in Europe. *Am J Clin Nutr* 106 (Suppl 6): 1655S–1662S.

Pavord, S., Daru, J., Prasannan, N. et al. (2020). UK guidelines on the management of iron deficiency in pregnancy. *Br J Haematol* 188: 819–830.

Peña-Rosas, J.P., De-Regil, L.M., Garcia-Casal, M.N., and Dowswell, T. (2015). Daily oral iron supplementation during pregnancy. *Cochrane Database Syst Rev* 2015 (7): CD004736.

van Santen S, Kroot JJ, Zijderveld G, et al. (2013). The iron regulatory hormone hepcidin is decreased in pregnancy: a prospective longitudinal study. *Clin Chem Lab Med* 51:1395–1401.

World Health Organisation and Food and Agriculture Organisation of the United Nations (2002). Human Vitamin and Mineral Requirements, Chapter 13 Iron.

14

Iron Deficiency in Gynaecology

Imo J. Akpan

Department of Medicine, Division of Haematology/Oncology, Columbia University Irving Medical Center, New York, NY, USA

Introduction

Abnormal uterine bleeding (AUB) is a major cause of iron deficiency (ID) in gynaecology. In women of reproductive age, heavy menstrual bleeding (HMB) affects at least 18–38% of this population. Patients with HMB and severe ID or iron deficiency anaemia (IDA) can have significant detriment to their quality of life.

Causes of Heavy Menstrual Bleeding

AUB includes atypical menstrual and intermenstrual bleeding. It is caused by uterine abnormalities such as fibroids (Figure 14.1), polyps, adenomyosis, malignancy, coagulopathy, ovulatory dysfunction and iatrogenic causes.

Definition of Heavy Menstrual Bleeding

HMB is one type of AUB and is defined as menstrual loss of more than 80 mLs per period cycle. The gold standard of extracting haematin from the sanitary product is not practical. A low ferritin level, clots 2.5 cm diameter and 'flooding' which means changing the pad or tampon every hour, is usually sufficient to conclude HMB.

Prevention of Iron Deficiency in Gynaecology

The mainstay of prevention of ID in this population includes measures to minimise and correct the underlying cause of the HMB. A balanced diet with adequate iron intake should also be recommended.

Iron in Clinical Practice, First Edition. Edited by Sue Pavord and Noemi Roy.
© 2025 John Wiley & Sons Ltd. Published 2025 by John Wiley & Sons Ltd.
Companion website: www.wiley.com/go/medicine5e

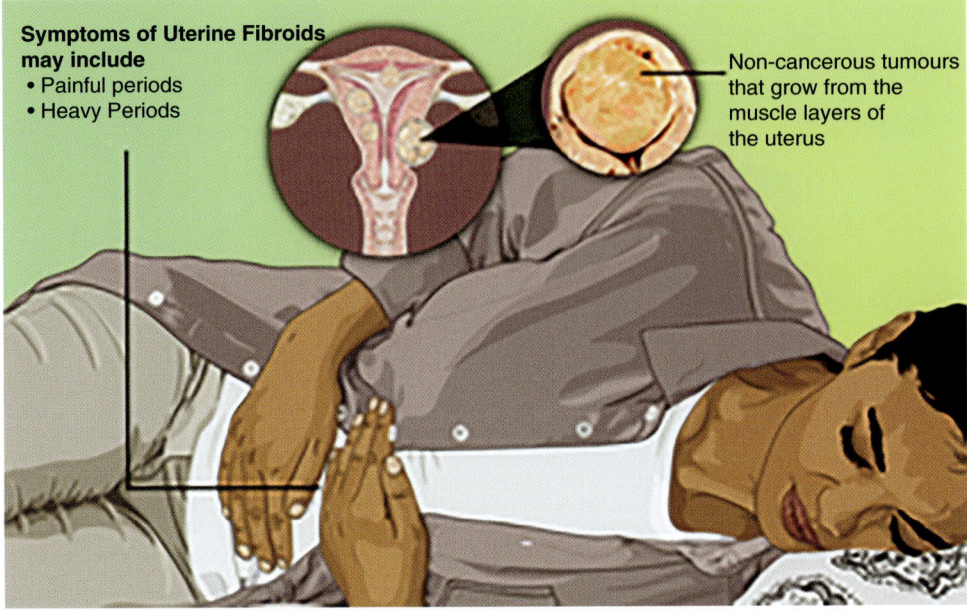

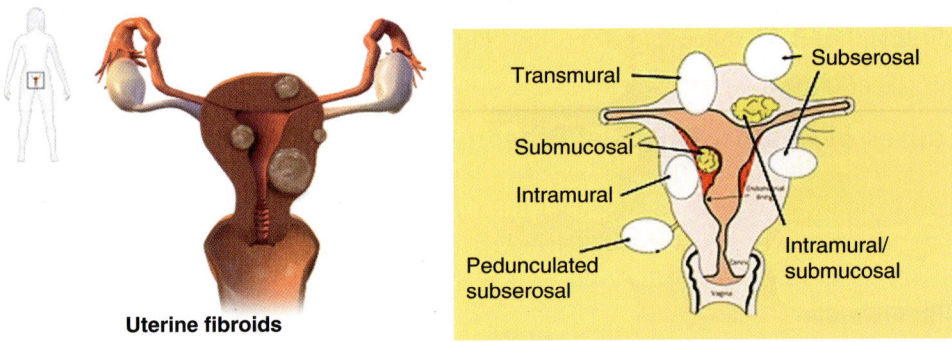

Figure 14.1 Fibroids.

Investigation of Heavy Menstrual Bleeding

Management requires a comprehensive patient and family history, physical examination and thorough review of medications. A transabdominal and transvaginal ultrasound may be indicated to assess for fibroids, cysts and adenomyosis. Advanced imaging is required when malignancy is suspected or better characterisation of structural uterine abnormalities is needed.

Underlying bleeding disorders should be considered and a detailed bleeding history taken or use of a bleeding assessment tool. If these are suggestive, investigations include prothrombin time, activated partial thromboplastin time, von Willebrand profile and coagulation factors. Extended studies, such as platelet function tests, may be indicated to make a final diagnosis of some bleeding disorders.

Management of Heavy Menstrual Bleeding

Hormonal contraception is an important part of initial management but may be insufficient or inappropriate in some patients. In other cases, a multidisciplinary team can be invaluable, including a haematologist, endocrinologist, interventional radiologist, surgeon and family physician.

Hormonal Preparations

These include combined hormonal contraception (CHC), oestrogen and progesterone-only or progestin-only options (Figure 14.2). The CHC increases the risk of thrombosis about 4–8 fold and should be avoided in patients with a history of thrombosis unless they are on continued anticoagulation. In patients with von Willebrand disease, CHCs have the added advantage of raising von Willebrand and Factor VIII levels. In some patients, the progesterone intrauterine device (IUD) can minimise or even stop the flow of menstrual bleeding completely. The first 4–6 weeks after IUD insertion can be associated with increased bleeding.

Anticoagulation Modification

In women on anticoagulation for venous thromboembolic disease or other indications, the incidence of HMB is 22–70%. Sometimes this is manageable for a short duration; however, patients who require indefinite anticoagulation can benefit from modification of treatment.

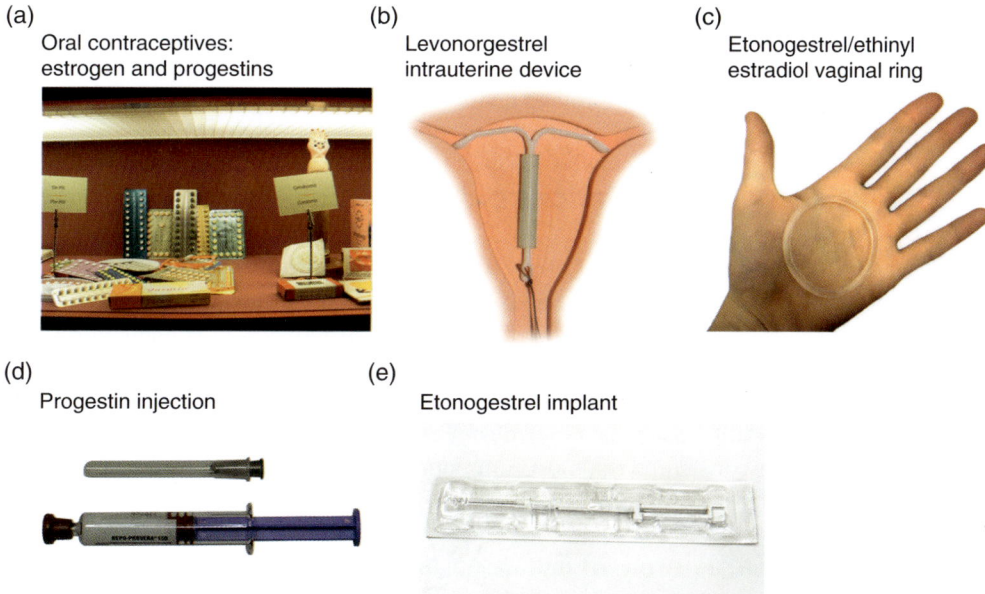

(a) Oral contraceptives: estrogen and progestins

(b) Levonorgestrel intrauterine device

(c) Etonogestrel/ethinyl estradiol vaginal ring

(d) Progestin injection

(e) Etonogestrel implant

Figure 14.2 Hormonal management of heavy menstrual bleeding. *Sources:* (a) Ryan Somma / Flickr / CC BY SA 2.0. (b) Hic et nunc / Wikimedia Commons / Public domain. (c) Sakky / Wikimedia Commons / Public domain. (d, e) Ciell / Wikimedia Commons / CC BY SA 2.5.

Whenever possible, the risks and benefits of stopping anticoagulation should be reassessed and anticoagulation must be stopped once it is no longer needed. For patients who need extended or indefinite anticoagulation, a lower prophylactic dose of the anticoagulant may be preferred, to balance a reduction in HMB without increasing thrombotic risk. Studies suggest that dabigatran causes less HMB compared to other direct oral anticoagulants.

Haemostatic Agents

Use of antifibrinolytic therapy (tranexamic acid and aminocaproic acid) during menstruation is also an option and is often prescribed for the first 2–3 days of each period, when bleeding is heaviest. Such use does not increase the risk of thrombosis in patients with HMB. Desmopressin intranasal spray or injection can be used in patients with von Willebrand disease, low factor VIII level or platelet dysfunction, but cautiously as it can lead to hyponatraemia and seizures (Figure 14.3). For patients with severe factor deficiencies, appropriate factor replacement such as a VWF/FVIII concentrate may be indicated.

Surgical Management

Surgical options include dilation and curettage, endometrial ablation, myomectomy and uterine artery embolisation for patients with fibroids. Whilst these options can be effective in some patients, some require repeat procedures and others may eventually need and opt for the only definitive intervention, hysterectomy. This can be an option in patients who no longer desire fertility, have a malignancy or whose symptoms have been difficult to manage with the non-definitive options. It is associated with surgical complications such as infection, bleeding and thrombosis. Hysterectomy-specific complications also include urinary and sexual issues. Nonetheless, a randomised study showed that hysterectomy was superior to medical management in improving quality of life (Figure 14.3).

Iron Deficiency and Iron Deficiency Anaemia in Gynaecology

Non-anaemic ID is underdiagnosed especially as HMB is underreported. Reasons for underreporting include a lack of awareness, aversion to discussion of menstruation by healthcare providers and variability in reporting of HMB. About 50% of women with HMB present to a provider for care and many do not receive adequate treatment. In addition to HMB, ID can be worsened by patients with a history of frequent blood donation, bariatric surgery or comorbidities such as renal dysfunction and inflammatory bowel disease (Table 14.1). HMB is considered the most common cause of IDA across the globe.

Impact of Iron Deficiency in Gynaecology

As ID leads to mobilisation of iron from ferritin, iron enzymes and proteins, the symptoms of ID are widespread and include fatigue, cognitive impairment, muscle weakness and restless legs. Other symptoms include alopecia and pica. It is important to screen for ID in

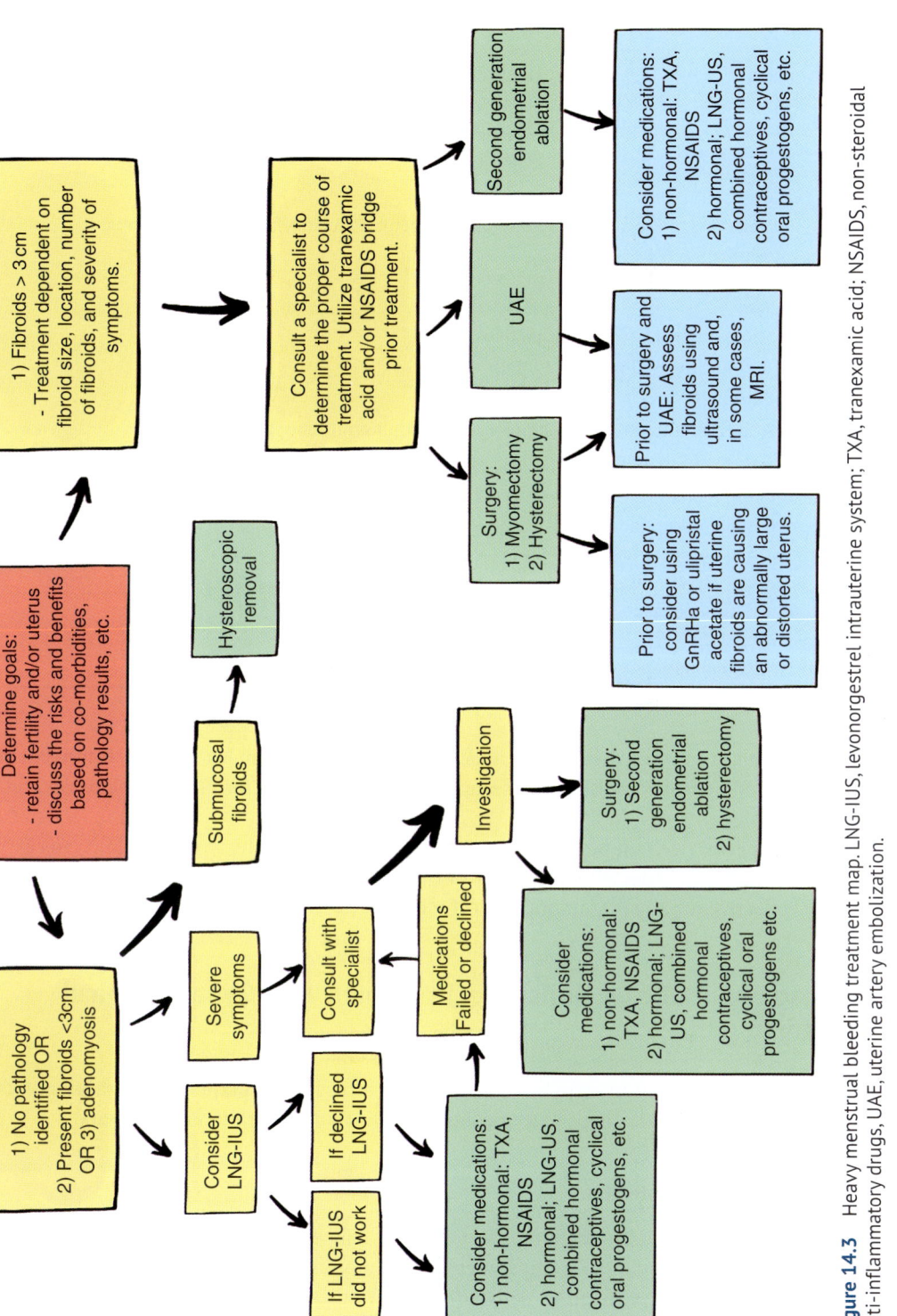

Figure 14.3 Heavy menstrual bleeding treatment map. LNG-IUS, levonorgestrel intrauterine system; TXA, tranexamic acid; NSAIDS, non-steroidal anti-inflammatory drugs, UAE, uterine artery embolization.

Table 14.1 Risks for iron deficiency in gynaecology.

Abnormal uterine bleeding/heavy menstrual bleeding

Structural causes:

Fibroids, endometriosis and malignancy

Bleeding disorder:

Inherited

Platelet function disorder and coagulation factor deficiency most commonly von Willebrand disease

Hereditary haemorrhagic telangiectasia

Acquired

Anticoagulation use and antiplatelet therapy

Trauma to the vaginal area

Ovulatory disorder

Hormonal disorder: thyroid disorder, polycystic ovarian syndrome (PCOS)

Conditions that worsen iron deficiency in gynaecology

Decreased iron intake (vegetarian/vegan diet)

Decreased iron absorption

History of bariatric surgery

Inflammatory bowel disease

Chronic kidney disease

Coeliac disease

Frequent blood donation

---

these patients even when they are not anaemic. Diagnosing ID can lead to early intervention with oral and IV iron supplementation and minimise the need for blood transfusion and/or in extreme cases hospitalisation.

Overall ID and IDA can negatively impact quality of life and the women's ability to carry out their daily activities. Absenteeism from work as a result of severe fatigue also has a larger collective negative economic impact on the society.

Management of Iron Deficiency in Women with Gynaecological Bleeding

Dietary supplementation with iron-rich food sources is inadequate for treatment of established ID in gynaecology, and oral and IV iron supplementation is necessary.

Oral Iron Supplementation

Oral iron supplementation should be initiated but may not be sufficient in cases of severe IDA and ongoing blood loss. Often women are not monitored closely to assess for adequate response and may be struggling with fatigue and other symptoms for several weeks or months before being considered for IV iron.

Parenteral Iron Supplementation

This is often underutilised but in women who are intolerant to oral iron, require rapid correction of iron stores or who are very severely iron deficient, IV iron supplementations may be necessary. Similarly, it is needed in women with malabsorption conditions or inflammatory disease where high hepcidin levels impair intestinal absorption of iron (Table 14.1). For women requiring surgical intervention, ID should be sought for and corrected preoperatively, with IV iron if there is insufficient time for oral iron to be effective. In women scheduled for hysterectomy to address HMB, about 23% were found to be anaemic. An improvement in preoperative haemoglobin levels reduces the need for blood transfusion and improves surgical outcomes.

Blood Transfusion

As anaemia is the end point of ID, some women with severe IDA with haemoglobin <70 g/L and profound symptoms may require blood transfusion. As ID is a chronic state, with time for endogenous red cell and cardiovascular compensatory mechanisms, blood transfusion is seldom necessary but one unit of red cells along with IV iron can be given if needed. In order to avoid transfusion, early evaluation and correction of ID is paramount.

Bibliography

Bofill, R.M., Lethaby, A., and Jordan, V. (2020). Progestogen-releasing intrauterine systems for heavy menstrual bleeding. *Cochrane Database Syst Rev* 6 (6): CD002126.

Gray, B., Floyd, S., and James, A.H. (2018). Contraceptive management for women who are at high risk of thrombosis. *Clin Obstet Gynecol* 61 (2): 243–249.

James, A.H. (2016). Heavy menstrual bleeding: work-up and management. *Hematology Am Soc Hematol Educ Program* 2016 (1): 236–242.

Mansour, D., Hofmann, A., and Gemzell-Danielsson, K. (2021). A review of clinical guidelines on the management of iron deficiency and iron-deficiency anemia in women with heavy menstrual bleeding. *Adv Ther* 38 (1): 201–225.

Munro, M.G., Mast, A.E., Powers, J.M. et al. (2023). The relationship between heavy menstrual bleeding, iron deficiency, and iron deficiency anemia. *Am J Obstet Gynecol* 229 (1): 1–9.

Tang, C., King, K., Ross, B., and Hamad, N. (2022). Iron deficiency in women: clearing the rust of silence. *Lancet Haematol* 9: e247–e248.

15

Iron Deficiency in Orthopaedics

Antony Palmer

Department of Surgery, Nuffield Orthopaedic Hospital, Oxford University Hospitals NHS Foundation Trust, Oxford, UK

Introduction

One-third of patients have anaemia prior to orthopaedic surgery. The prevalence is higher in some patient groups, such as those who sustained a neck of femur fracture. In two-thirds of cases, the cause of the anaemia is iron deficiency (ID), acknowledging that the diagnostic criteria for both anaemia and ID vary widely. Preoperative anaemia increases the likelihood of allogeneic blood transfusion and the associated risks of perioperative complications. There is a dose–response relationship between blood transfusion and surgical site infection in hip and knee arthroplasty. Patients with ID anaemia also have an increased length of postoperative stay and higher costs following orthopaedic surgery. Studies into how different therapeutic iron formulations are best absorbed and utilised in a variety of clinical scenarios can be used to guide how and when iron is best used in the perioperative period to prevent and/or treat anaemia and improve patient outcomes.

Diagnosis

When orthopaedic surgery is planned, anaemia should be diagnosed at the earliest opportunity in the patient pathway, to permit sufficient time to investigate and optimise iron status. Ideally this process should be initiated as soon as surgical intervention is under consideration, and not at a preoperative assessment a few weeks prior to surgery. Target haemoglobin (Hb) should be 130 g/L in males and females. Circulating volume is lower in females, and therefore blood losses are proportionally higher. There is significant variation in practice for the laboratory diagnosis of ID, and ferritin thresholds range from <30 ug/L to >100 ug/L in the presence of inflammation. Ferritin <30 ug/L or transferrin saturation <20% strongly suggests ID.

Iron in Clinical Practice, First Edition. Edited by Sue Pavord and Noemi Roy.
© 2025 John Wiley & Sons Ltd. Published 2025 by John Wiley & Sons Ltd.
Companion website: www.wiley.com/go/medicine5e

Aetiology of Iron Deficiency

The aetiology of anaemia and ID varies between different orthopaedic populations. Patients may be iron deficient due to pre-existing medical conditions that may reduce iron absorption such as chronic inflammation or gastrointestinal pathology. These aetiologies are often prevalent within patient cohorts with inflammatory arthritis. There may also be poor dietary intake or chronic bleeding, such as menstruation. These etiologies are often prevalent within cohorts of young females undergoing scoliosis surgery. Patients sustaining neck of femur fractures are often frail with multiple comorbidities, including chronic renal failure. It is important to exclude undiagnosed malignancy as a cause of anaemia, and referral to gastroenterology may be appropriate. The development of an algorithm for the investigation and treatment of perioperative anaemia requires input from an extended multidisciplinary team and will differ between institutions. There are many guidelines available that outline best care.

Preoperative Treatment of Iron Deficiency Anaemia

Oral iron supplementation is the mainstay of treatment for ID anaemia prior to elective orthopaedic surgery. In the absence of inflammation (CRP <5 mg/L), oral iron supplementation is an effective treatment. High dose oral iron therapy has a high rate of gastrointestinal side effects, poor compliance and can stimulate hepcidin release, reducing iron absorption. Low dose therapy taken on alternate days is better tolerated and more effective. Iron supplementation should be commenced shortly after diagnosis, and improvements in Hb are usually seen within 4 weeks.

Oral iron supplementation is less effective in the presence of inflammation, such as inflammatory arthritis, when intravenous iron therapy should be considered. Intravenous iron increases Hb faster than oral iron, making it well suited for urgent surgery, such as procedures to treat malignancy. Patients who fail to respond to, or cannot tolerate, oral iron may also benefit from intravenous iron. Studies have shown an association between intravenous iron and infection, so it should be used with caution in patients with active infection. Other potential complications of intravenous iron are anaphylaxis, hypophosphataemia and venous extravasation.

There is inadequate time to treat ID prior to emergency surgery; however, iron supplementation should be considered in the postoperative period. Postoperatively, patients will experience systemic inflammation and intravenous iron therapy is more likely to be effective than oral iron. Orthopaedic patients may have severe anaemia in the postoperative period. Intravenous iron may represent an alternative to allogeneic blood transfusion, and addressing postoperative anaemia is particularly important when further surgery is planned. Potential complications of intravenous iron infusion are likely outweighed by complications associated with allogeneic blood transfusion.

Patient Outcomes

The diagnosis and treatment of preoperative anaemia reduce the risk of perioperative blood transfusion in orthopaedic surgery. For a given blood loss, a higher starting Hb will make reaching a transfusion threshold less likely, and optimising anaemia is a key metric in delivering best care. It may be appropriate to postpone surgery to allow time to optimise anaemia, with the goal of reducing the risk or volume of transfusion and improving patient outcomes.

Cohort studies, most frequently of patients undergoing hip and knee replacement, demonstrate that treating preoperative ID anaemia reduces the risk of transfusion, readmission, critical care admission, prolonged length of stay and cost. However, randomised controlled trials of preoperative iron supplementation do not replicate these findings and often show no benefit in patient outcomes. The results of these trials prompt reassessment of our approach to perioperative anaemia. Trial limitations include wide inclusion criteria and inadequate power for subgroup analyses, or it may be that anaemia represents a marker of morbidity rather than a modifiable risk factor for adverse outcomes. Further research is required in this field. Current guidelines and quality standards emphasise the important of optimising preoperative anaemia.

Understanding the aetiology of anaemia is important to tailor treatment, and the benefits of treatment may be procedure specific. Modern patient blood management strategies have reduced intraoperative blood losses and the demand for blood (Figure 15.1). Therefore, preoperative anaemia may not translate to perioperative blood transfusions, and it is likely that immunomodulation from allogeneic blood is an important cause of adverse outcomes. However, there are other health benefits to diagnosing and treating preoperative anaemia, and oral iron supplementation is inexpensive and with an alternate-day dosing regimen, well tolerated with few adverse events.

	Pillars of patient blood management		
	Optimize erythropoiesis	Minimize blood loss	Manage anaemia
Pre-op	Diagnose, investigate, and treat the cause of the anaemia at the earliest opportunity	Identify, discuss, and manage antiplatelet agents and anticoagulants appropriately	Develop patient-specific transfusion plan if high risk of major hemorrhage or limited allogeneic blood available
Intra-op	Schedule surgery when hemoglobin optimized. If anemic, consider staging the surgery, for example unilateral rather than bilateral	Use tranexamic acid, cell salvage, and careful surgical techniques to limit blood loss at surgery	Use restrictive transfusion thresholds
Post-op	Consider most appropriate post-op treatment of anaemia, such as intravenous iron	Monitor for post-op bleeding that may be overt or hidden. Manage antiplatelet agents and anticoagulants	Use restrictive transfusion thresholds

The darker boxes represent the perioperative stage most applicable to the pillar of patient blood management

Figure 15.1 Pillars of patient blood management in orthopaedic surgery.

Iron Deficiency Without Anaemia

Preoperative ID is prevalent, and patients may not have anaemia. However, following hip and knee arthroplasty surgery, more than three-quarters of patients will have anaemia on discharge from hospital. Preoperative replacement of iron in those with non-anaemia ID reduces the risk of allogeneic blood transfusion. However, as yet, this intervention has not been shown to improve surgical outcomes and at present there is insufficient evidence to support routine treatment of preoperative ID without anaemia.

Bibliography

Muñoz, M., Acheson, A.G., Auerbach, M. et al. (2017). International consensus statement on the peri-operative management of anaemia and iron deficiency. *Anaesthesia* 72 (2): 233–247.

Palmer, A.J.R., Gagne, S., Fergusson, D. et al. (2020). Blood management for elective orthopaedic surgery. *J Bone Joint Surg Am* 102 (17): 1552–1564.

Scrimshire, A.B., Booth, A., Fairhurst, C. et al. (2020). Preoperative iron treatment in anaemic patients undergoing elective total hip or knee arthroplasty: a systematic review and meta-analysis. *BMJ Open* 10 (10): e036592.

Shah, A., Palmer, A.J.R., and Klein, A.A. (2020). Strategies to minimize intraoperative blood loss during major surgery. *Br J Surg* 107 (2): e26–e38.

Shah, A.A., Donovan, K., Seeley, C. et al. (2021). Risk of infection associated with administration of intravenous iron: a systematic review and meta-analysis. *JAMA Netw Open* 4 (11): e2133935.

16

Iron Deficiency in Intensive Care

Akshay Shah[1,2]

[1] Nuffield Department of Clinical Neurosciences, University of Oxford, Oxford University Hospitals NHS Foundation Trust, Oxford, UK
[2] Department of Anaesthesia, Hammersmith Hospital, Imperial College Healthcare NHS Trust, London, UK

Introduction

Every year around 260,000 adults are admitted to UK intensive care units (ICUs). Historical data, using conventional tests of iron status, report that the incidence of iron deficiency at the time of ICU admission is 35%, although the true estimate is likely to be higher.

Iron Homeostasis in Critical Illness

In health, systemic iron levels are finely balanced between supply and demand. Critical illness triggers an inflammatory response that results in early, profound and sometimes persistent changes in iron homeostasis. Inflammation upregulates acute phase proteins such as ferritin and lactoferrin that bind free iron with a greater affinity than transferrin – the circulating iron transporter and negative acute phase reactant, which results in systemic hypoferraemia (Figure 16.1). Inflammatory cytokines, in particular interleukin (IL)-6, stimulate hepatocytes to produce the key iron regulatory hormone – hepcidin. Hepcidin expression results in internalisation and degradation of ferroportin – the only known mammalian exporter of iron, which blocks release of iron from macrophages and absorption of iron by duodenal enterocytes (Chapter 2).

These processes are part of a highly conserved evolutionary response designed to limit free (or non-transferrin bound) iron for invading pathogens, particularly iron-dependent extracellular organisms that could otherwise cause severe infection (Chapter 3). Other cytokines such as tumour necrosis factor-α, IL-1 and IL-10 reduce duodenal iron absorption and facilitate iron acquisition macrophages through transferrin-receptor mediated endocytosis, but these mechanisms are poorly characterised to date.

Iron in Clinical Practice, First Edition. Edited by Sue Pavord and Noemi Roy.
© 2025 John Wiley & Sons Ltd. Published 2025 by John Wiley & Sons Ltd.
Companion website: www.wiley.com/go/medicine5e

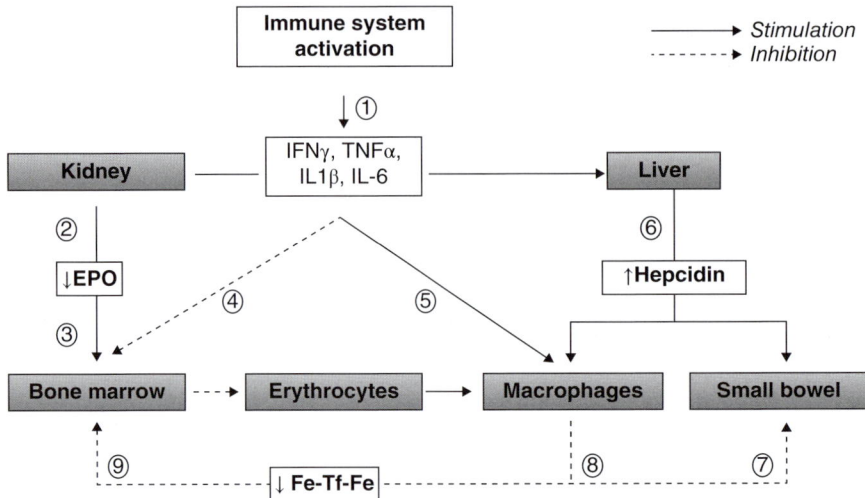

Figure 16.1 Iron homeostasis in critically ill patients. *Source:* Muñoz et al. (2017) / John Wiley & Sons.

Table 16.1 Definitions, laboratory characteristics and potential treatment strategies of stages of iron deficiency seen in intensive care.

Iron status	Definition	Laboratory findings	Iron therapy strategies
True/absolute iron deficiency	Depletion of body iron stores, which are inadequate to maintain erythropoiesis	Ferritin <30 µg/L or Tsat <20% and/or CHr <30 pg, Hb > 130 g/L, Low hepcidin	Oral iron; IV iron if not taking oral medication
Iron-deficiency anaemia	Reduced Hb and erythrocytes due to insufficient iron availability	Hb < 130 g/L, ferritin <30 µg/L or Tsat <20% and/or CHr 30 pg, low hepcidin	Oral iron, IV iron if not taking oral medication or rapid correction required
Functional iron deficiency	Insufficient mobilisation of iron stores due to increased demands, despite adequate iron stores	Ferritin >100 µg/L and Tsat <20% and/or CHr ≥30 pg, Possibly raised CRP Variable hepcidin	IV iron; consider oral iron if low disease activity or inflammatory burden
Iron sequestration / iron-restricted erythropoiesis	Reduced supply of iron to meet erythropoietic requirements	Ferritin 30–100 µg/L, Tsat <20%, CRP >5 mg/L or eGFR <60 mL/min Raised hepcidin	IV iron; consider erythropoietin

CHr, Reticulocyte haemoglobin content; CRP, C-reactive protein; eGFR, estimated glomerular filtration rate; Hb, haemoglobin; IV, intravenous; Tsat, percent transferrin saturation.
Source: Adapted from Benson et al. (2021).

Diagnosing Iron Deficiency in Critical Illness

Characterising the type of iron deficiency (functional versus absolute) in critical illness is challenging as inflammation confounds the interpretation of common tests of iron status, including ferritin and percent transferrin saturation (Tsat). One approach has been to alter the thresholds of the results of these tests to account for the acute phase response, often in combination with C-reactive protein (CRP) (Table 16.1). The World Health Organisation recommends that a ferritin cut-off of 70 mcg/L may be indicative of iron deficiency in adults with coexisting infection or inflammation. However, validation of these thresholds against a gold standard of iron deficiency in critically ill patients is lacking.

Serum hepcidin may be a more reliable measure of iron status even in the presence of inflammation, whilst also being able to identify which patients may benefit from iron therapy. Large validation studies using accurate, clinically available hepcidin assays are required. Other potentially useful tests include soluble transferrin receptor – a marker of tissue iron need, and reticulocyte haemoglobin content – a measure of the amount of iron available for haemoglobin production in the bone marrow.

Clinical Implications of Iron Deficiency in Intensive Care Unit

Iron is essential for haemoglobin synthesis, cell growth, neurotransmission, immunity and cardiopulmonary function. Many cellular proteins and enzymes also require iron to function. Disturbances in iron homeostasis are of prognostic significance in critically ill patients in a U-shaped relationship (Figure 16.2).

High serum iron and percent Tsat are associated with increased mortality in critically ill patients admitted with sepsis. Conversely, hypoferraemia is associated with worsening hypoxemia, impaired immune responses to infection and increased risk of bloodstream

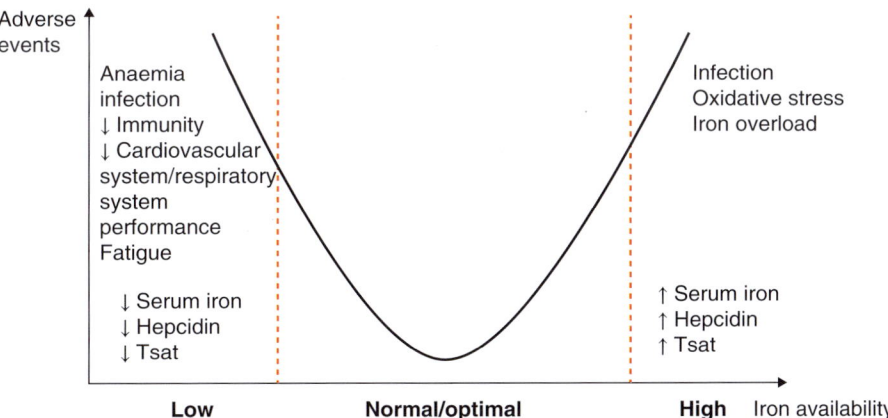

Figure 16.2 Complications of altered iron status in critically ill patients. *Source:* Adapted from Litton and Lim (2019).

infection. Low hepcidin levels (<20 ng/ml) at ICU discharge is associated with increased one-year mortality and poor physical recovery.

The persistent state of iron restriction inevitably leads to the development of anaemia. Anaemia is independently associated with poor short- and long-term outcomes, and it remains the most common indication for a red blood cell transfusion in critically ill patients.

Patient Blood Management in Intensive Care

Red cell transfusion is the current mainstay of treating anaemia in critically ill patients. Even though transfusion practice has moved towards a more restrictive approach over the past two decades, one in four patients still receive a red cell transfusion during their ICU admission. With the advances in our understanding of iron homeostasis and erythropoiesis in critical illness, there has been increasing use of alternative strategies such as iron therapy to treat anaemia, reduce red cell transfusion requirements and improve patient outcomes.

Intravenous Iron in Intensive Care

Intravenous iron can bypass the 'hepcidin block' caused by inflammation and is an efficacious way for treating iron deficiency in intensive care patients (see Chapter 6).

Current concerns in critically ill patients include the risk of hypophosphataemia, particularly with ferric carboxymaltose, although the clinical significance after a single infusion is unclear. Another concern has been the risk of precipitating or exacerbating infection. Subgroup analysis of critically ill patients has not so far demonstrated increased risk of infection associated with intravenous iron therapy, but it should be avoided where there is active bacteraemia.

Systematic reviews and small trials of intravenous iron, such as single-dose 1000 mg ferric carboxymaltose at ICU discharge, have demonstrated improvements in haemoglobin that may possibly translate into better outcomes, with no safety concerns. The relative risks and benefits of intravenous iron likely depend on the timing of administration, for example, the recovery phase of critical illness may be a more suitable timepoint as there is a wider therapeutic window and the benefits may outweigh the risks. However, large confirmatory trials are warranted.

Concomitant Therapies for Anaemia Management in Intensive Care

Recombinant erythropoietin (rHuEPO) in combination with intravenous iron is an attractive, biologically plausible treatment option for the anaemia of inflammation that accompanies critical illness. rHuEPO stimulates erythropoiesis but also suppresses hepcidin production through upregulation of erythroferrone and possibly IL-6 suppression. Prolyl hydroxylase inhibitors stimulate production of endogenous EPO and may also act on intestinal mucosa to increase iron absorption. They are approved for use for treating anaemia in patients with chronic kidney disease requiring dialysis. Phase I/II trials are currently ongoing, evaluating various monoclonal antibodies and nucleotides that reduce hepcidin concentrations and reverse hypoferraemia. Subsets of critically ill patients may benefit from such therapies in the future.

Bibliography

Benson, C.S., Shah, A., Stanworth, S.J. et al. (2021). The effect of iron deficiency and anaemia on women's health. *Anaesthesia* 76 (S4): 84–95. https://doi.org/10.1111/anae.15405.

Geneen, L.J., Kimber, C., Doree, C. et al. (2022). Efficacy and safety of intravenous iron therapy for treating anaemia in critically ill adults: a rapid systematic review with meta-analysis. *Transfus Med Rev* 36 (2): 97–106.

Lasocki, S., Lefebvre, T., Mayeur, C. et al. (2018). Iron deficiency diagnosed using hepcidin on critical care discharge is an independent risk factor for death and poor quality of life at one year: an observational prospective study on 1161 patients. *Crit Care* 22 (1): 314.

Litton, E., French, C., Herschtal, A. et al. (2023). Iron and erythropoietin to heal and recover after intensive care (ITHRIVE): a pilot randomised clinical trial. *Crit Care Resusc* 25 (4): 201–206.

Litton, E. and Lim, J. (2019). Iron metabolism: an emerging therapeutic target in critical illness. *Crit Care* 23 (1): 81. https://doi.org/10.1186/s13054-019-2373-1.

Munoz M, Acheson AG, Auerbach M, et al. International consensus statement on the perioperative management of anaemia and iron deficiency. *Anaesthesia* 2017;72(2):233–247. https://doi.org/10.1111/anae.13773

Shah, A., Chester-Jones, M., Dutton, S.J. et al. (2022). Intravenous iron to treat anaemia following critical care: a multicentre feasibility randomised trial. *Br J Anaesth* 128 (2): 272–282.

Shah, A., Frost, J.N., Aaron, L. et al. (2020). Systemic hypoferremia and severity of hypoxemic respiratory failure in COVID-19. *Crit Care* 24 (1): 320.

Tacke, F., Nuraldeen, R., Koch, A. et al. (2016). Iron parameters determine the prognosis of critically ill patients. *Crit Care Med* 44 (6): 1049–1058.

17

Iron Deficiency in Medical Oncology

Sue Pavord

Department of Haematology, Oxford University Hospitals NHS Foundation Trust, Oxford, UK

Introduction

Anaemia is highly prevalent in cancer patients and correlates with poor performance status and quality of life. The causes of anaemia are multifactorial, but iron deficiency (ID) is a significant contributor in approximately half of patients with solid tumours and haematological malignancy, with a roughly equal split of absolute and functional ID.

Causes of Anaemia in Patients with Cancer

There are many confounding factors contributing to anaemia in oncology patients. Included in this are potential deficiencies of iron, B12, folate, and other vitamins, due to anorexia or malabsorption; chemotherapy-induced anaemia, including off-target effects of specific agents such as tyrosine kinase inhibitors and monoclonal antibodies; renal anaemia from inadequate erythropoietin production; and bone marrow infiltration. However, these factors may not be present and anaemia arises from both the impaired erythropoietic activity and disturbed iron homeostasis which occur with increased inflammatory cytokines due to the underlying cancer and/or toxicity of local or systemic anticancer therapy (SACT). Elevated hepcidin levels with internalisation of ferroportin give rise to a functional ID with iron trapped within the intestinal cells, macrophages and hepatocytes (see Chapter 2). ID is defined as a lack of available iron for cellular functions and in cancer patients, it may be a functional ID, absolute ID or a combination of both.

Iron in Clinical Practice, First Edition. Edited by Sue Pavord and Noemi Roy.
© 2025 John Wiley & Sons Ltd. Published 2025 by John Wiley & Sons Ltd.
Companion website: www.wiley.com/go/medicine5e

Diagnosis of Iron Deficiency in Patients with Cancer

Ferritin is an acute phase reactant, whose expression is elevated by tumour necrosis factor TNF-α. Elevated ferritin may in fact reflect disease severity, rather than replete iron status. Therefore, for patients with cancer, a higher threshold of 100 mcg/L is taken to distinguish between absolute and functional ID.

The percent transferrin saturation (TSAT) is also influenced by inflammation; transferrin is the plasma iron chaperone, but is an acute negative phase protein, as its production is inhibited by TNF-α. Thus, the lower percent TSAT seen in ID may be masked by the fall in total transferrin levels – transferrin concentration being the denominator in calculating TSAT.

With these limitations in mind, absolute ID is defined as TSAT <20% and serum ferritin <100 mcg/L and functional ID as TSAT <20% and serum ferritin >100 mcg/L.

Other laboratory parameters usually suggestive of ID, such as red cell hypochromia and microcytosis, are less helpful in the presence of cancer and chronic inflammation.

Biomarkers such as a low cellular haemoglobin content in reticulocytes (RetHe < 28 pg) and an increased percentage of hypochromic red cells of >5% can reflect both absolute and functional ID. Soluble transferrin receptor (sTfR) value is increased in patients with absolute ID and usually within normal limits or low in functional ID. It has been observed to increase with erythropoiesis stimulating treatment (ESA) and reduce following chemotherapy.

Management of Anaemia in Patients with Cancer

The major aims of anaemia management are the reduction or resolution of anaemia symptoms, particularly fatigue, and an improved quality of life. The underlying cause(s) should be established to ensure targeted and appropriate treatment, with the minimum invasive treatment that corrects the underlying causes and proves to be safe.

In those identified with ID, oral iron may be attempted if serum ferritin is <30 mcg/L and there is no nausea or anorexia. Counselling about correct administration is important to ensure optimal absorption and minimal side effects (see Chapter 6).

For patients with inflammatory conditions (C-reactive protein >5 mg/L) and consequential impaired absorption, intravenous iron is required.

As iron is required for every cell in the body, including tumour cells, this potentially raises concern that intravenous iron could lead to tumour progression; however, this has not been borne out by clinical evidence, although longer-term follow up is required.

Erythropoiesis Stimulating Agents

If anaemia persists despite normal iron status, B12 and folate, treatment with an ESAs can be considered for patients undergoing SACT who have symptomatic anaemia and haemoglobin <100 g/L. ESAs have been shown to increase haemoglobin levels and to reduce the need for blood transfusions in these patients. Studies have also confirmed reduced fatigue and improved quality of life with ESAs used in this setting. The minimally effective dose should be used, to avoid increased thrombotic events. Approximately 60% of patients respond and if there is no improvement after four weeks the ESA should be discontinued.

Blood Transfusion in Oncology

Blood transfusion has long been used as the mainstay of treatment of anaemia in cancer patients but is associated with administrative errors leading to incorrect and incompatible blood transfusion and clinical risks including transfusion-associated circulatory overload, alloimmunisation, and longer-term iron accumulation with repeated transfusions.

Furthermore, in the setting of cancer surgery, large-scale population studies suggest independent associations between blood transfusions and increased mortality, morbidity and cancer recurrence.

Additionally, there have been concerns with the supply of blood in the United Kingdom. NHS Blood and Transplant have repeatedly issued warnings of low blood stocks. Therefore, focussing management on the identification and treatment of the underlying cause of anaemia is of paramount importance, to reduce need for allogeneic blood, not only for the benefit of the individual patient but also to conserve blood stocks.

Blood transfusion may be necessary in a non-bleeding patient if haemoglobin falls below 70 g/L, or 80 g/L for patients with cardiovascular disease, and there are symptoms of imped-ing normal activity. Use of these restrictive thresholds has been shown to lead to significant reductions in total and in-hospital mortality, rebleeding, acute coronary syndrome, pulmo-nary oedema and bacterial infections, compared with a more liberal strategy. Improvement in symptoms and haemoglobin is only transient as endogenous erythropoiesis is not stimu-lated and may be suppressed. Consent for transfusion should be obtained and only one unit given before clinical and laboratory reassessment.

Prevention of Anaemia in Patients with Cancer

Guidelines from the European Society for Medical Oncology (ESMO) recommend that all anae-mic patients referred for SACT have a %TSAT and serum ferritin checked. In ID, erythropoiesis is often prioritised and iron mobilised from stores and depleted from other cells before anaemia occurs. Therefore, even in non-anaemic individuals, iron status should be checked before SACT to identify and correct ID before ID anaemia develops. Local policies, in keeping with ESMO, for example, shown in Figure 17.1, are often welcome given the considerable saving on staff time with the avoidance of blood transfusion and not least the benefit to the patient.

Implementation of Local Policy

Blood transfusion is a nursing-intensive procedure, taking 3–4 hours in the outpatient setting and one that requires patients to attend for an additional blood test for crossmatching. In contrast, intravenous iron can be administered on the same day as chemotherapy, reducing

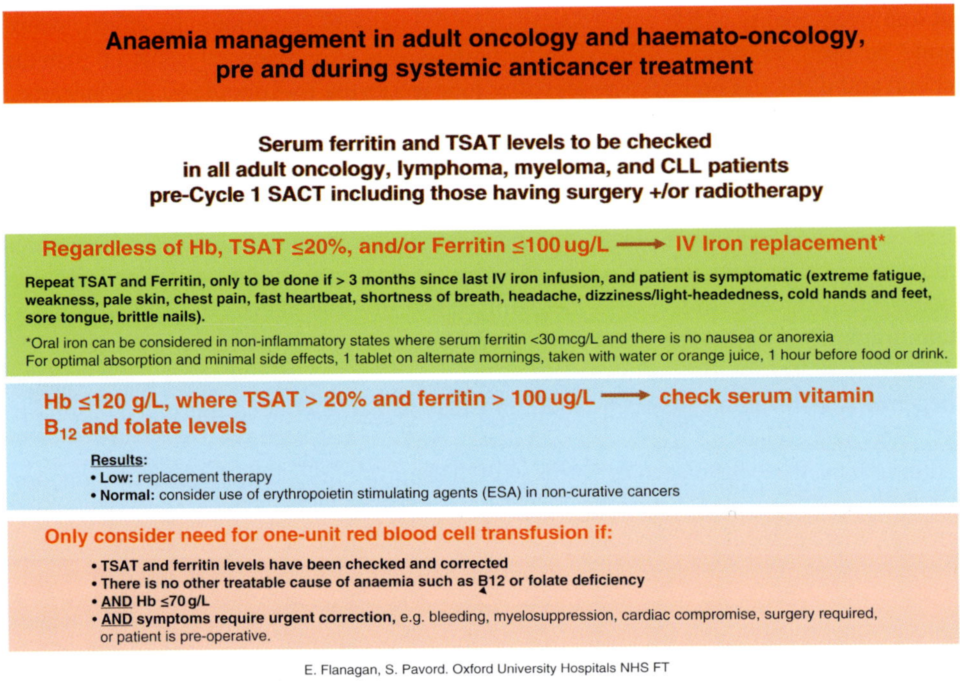

Figure 17.1 Local policy for management of anaemia in patients with cancer.

day-case admissions for patients and increasing capacity of the service. For patients receiving cardiotoxic anticancer therapy, same-day iron treatment is best avoided. Engagement of clinical teams and repeated audit cycles and education for medical, nursing and pharmacy staff are required to achieve successful outcomes and reduce the requirement for blood transfusion.

Novel Anti-anaemia Agents

Novel classes of anti-anaemic drugs are in development or being introduced. They include activin receptor ligand traps, hypoxia-inducible factor-prolyl hydroxylase inhibitors, and hepcidin antagonists. Whilst they are currently aimed at treatment for other causes of anaemia, cancer patients are likely to benefit from their use in the future.

Conclusion

In summary, anaemia is highly prevalent in medical oncology patients, with ID being a significant cause. The use of a local guideline to identify and treat ID in oncology patients receiving SACT results in a significant reduction in blood transfusion and associated risks and costs. Strategies such as these are paramount during such times of national blood

Table 17.1 Causes, presentation and management of iron deficiency in oncology patients.

Iron deficiency in oncology patients			
Causes	• Reduced availability • Poor diet • Malabsorption • Inflammation/chronic disease	• Increased loss • Bleeding and blood loss	• Increased demand • Increased erythropoiesis after chemotherapy

Symptoms	• Iron deficiency without anaemia
	  – Fatigue, brain fog, shortness of breath, palpitations, restless legs, hair loss and pica
	• Iron deficiency anaemia (additional)
	  – Weakness, dizziness, headache, cold extremities, pale skin, chest pain, mouth ulcers, slow/poor wound healing and tinnitus		

Complications	• Anaemia and associated complications, reduced quality of life and healthcare costs • Increased risk of blood transfusion		

Treatment options	• Iron supplementation
	  – Oral if absolute iron deficiency with low serum ferritin
	  – Intravenous if functional iron deficiency and normal serum ferritin		

shortages. Table 17.1 summarises the causes, symptoms, and current treatment options for ID in oncology patients. New antianaemic drugs on the horizon offer further hope for cancer patients.

Bibliography

Aapro, M., Beguin, Y., Bokemeyer, C. et al. (2018). Management of anaemia and iron deficiency in patients with cancer: ESMO Clinical Practice Guidelines. *Ann Oncol* 29 (Suppl 4): iv96–iv110.

Adams, A., Scheckel, B., Habsaoui, A. et al. (2022). Intravenous iron versus oral iron versus no iron with or without erythropoiesis- stimulating agents (ESA) for cancer patients with anaemia: a systematic review and network meta-analysis. *Cochrane Database Syst Rev* 6 (6): CD012633.

Bozzini, C., Busti, F., Marchi, G. et al. (2024). Anemia in patients receiving anticancer treatments: focus on novel therapeutic approaches. *Front Oncol* 14: 1380358. https://doi.org/10.3389/fonc.2024.1380358.

Carson, J.L., Stanworth, S.J., Guyatt, G. et al. (2023). Red blood cell transfusion: 2023 AABB international guidelines. *JAMA: J Am Med Assoc.* 330: 1892–1902. https://doi.org/10.1001/jama.2023.12914.

Gilreath, J.A. and Rodgers, G.M. (2020). How I treat cancer-associated anemia. *Blood* 136: 801–813. https://doi.org/10.1182/blood.2019004017.

Gluszak, C., de Vries-Brilland, M., Seegers, V. et al. (2022). Impact of iron-deficiency management on quality of life in patients with cancer: a prospective cohort study (CAMARA study). *Oncologist* 27: 328–333.

Part 3

Iron Overload

Part 3a

Causes of Iron Overload

18

Transfusional Iron Overload

Samah Babiker[1] and John Porter[2]

[1] *Evelina London Children's Hospital, St Thomas' Hospital, London, UK*
[2] *Department of Haematology, University College Hospital, London, UK*

Introduction

Unlike most animal species, human iron metabolism is conservative so that excess iron accumulated from repeated transfusions cannot be eliminated without phlebotomy or iron chelation. Transfusional iron overload (TIOL) is a potentially life-threatening condition that requires vigilant recognition, monitoring and proactive management. It predominantly affects patients receiving chronic or intermittent blood transfusions for congenital or acquired anaemia. If left unmanaged, the accumulation of excess iron in the body can result in serious endorgan damage by free radical induced tissue injury.

The Causes of Iron Overload and Influencing Factors

The consequences of repeated transfusions on iron distribution vary depending on the rates of blood transfusion and the duration of TIOL, as well as the underlying reasons for transfusion (Table 18.1). Regular top up blood transfusions results in a more rapid accumulation of iron compared to a slower accumulation with intermittent blood transfusion. Those on regular exchange transfusion programme may have a milder degree of iron overload or none at all, given the near iron-neutral nature of the procedure.

Pathophysiology and Effects of Transfusional Iron Loading on Body Iron Distribution

In healthy adults, body iron totals 40–50 mg/kg, mainly contained within red cell haemoglobin (30 mg/kg), with 20 mg/kg stored as ferritin and haemosiderin in hepatocytes or the macrophage system of the liver, spleen and bone marrow. Typically, a unit of blood (derived from about 470 mLs of donor blood) contains about 200 mg of iron and so for adults with

Iron in Clinical Practice, First Edition. Edited by Sue Pavord and Noemi Roy.
© 2025 John Wiley & Sons Ltd. Published 2025 by John Wiley & Sons Ltd.
Companion website: www.wiley.com/go/medicine5e

Table 18.1 Conditions at risk of transfusional iron overload.

Myelodysplastic syndrome

Aplastic anaemia

Red cell aplasia

Chronic myelofibrosis

Autoimmune haemolytic anaemia

Paroxysmal nocturnal haemoglobinuria

Systemic anticancer therapy

Bone marrow transplantation

Thalassaemia

Sideroblastic anaemia

Congenital dyserythropoietic anaemia

Pyruvate kinase deficiency

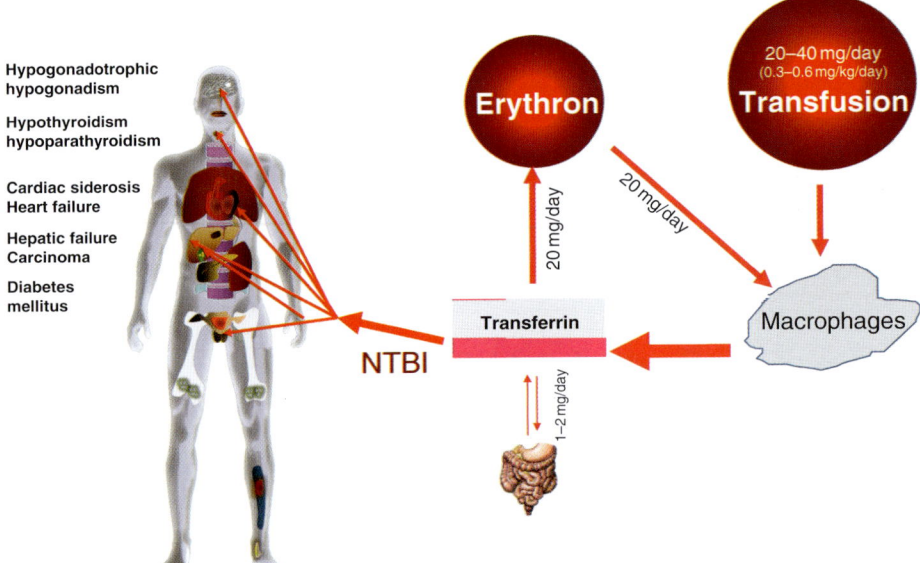

Figure 18.1 Distribution of iron overload. NTBI – non-transferrin-bound iron.

transfusion-dependent thalassaemia (TDT) the accumulation of iron from transfusion can be 10 g per year.

Iron from senescent transfused red cells is taken into macrophages of the spleen, liver and bone marrow, before haem catabolism and subsequent release of iron (II) through membrane ferroportin channels onto transferrin. Transferrin saturation increases with ongoing transfusion until non-transferrin-bound iron (NTBI) species are found in plasma (usually when >70% transferrin saturation). Transfusion iron loading then accumulates initially in liver hepatocytes as ferritin and hemosiderin (Figure 18.1).

With repeated transfusions, the liver iron concentration rises, and serum transferrin saturation increases, with a consequent rise in NTBI in the serum. NBTI is labile and highly reactive. It has the ability to catalyse the production of the free radicals through the Fenton reaction leading to cellular damage by oxidative stress. NTBI leads to a paradigm shift in iron distribution, with transferrin-independent iron uptake into myocardium and the endocrine system including the anterior pituitary.

Of both mechanistic interest and practical clinical importance, distribution of iron into the heart and endocrine system is less likely in transfusionally loaded sickle cell disease (SCD) than in TDT. Conversely, transfusion-dependent patients with Diamond Blackfan anaemia (DBA) can accumulate iron at a higher rate and those with congenital sideroblastic anaemia can accumulate iron in the heart faster than in the liver.

Rates of Transfusional Iron Overloading and Distribution in Different Diseases

TIOL is best described for thalassaemia major where transfusion typically begins within a few months of birth. The rate of transfusional iron loading varies with the underlying genetic mutations but ranges within 0.4 ± 0.11 mg/kg/day. If left untreated with chelation, liver iron concentration exceeds 15–20 mg/g dry weight within 10 years, exceeding the threshold for iron uptake into myocardium.

Transfusion in SCD is usually aimed at preventing complications of sickling more than correcting the anaemia itself. Severe iron overload therefore is less likely, particularly if red cell exchanges are performed rather than top ups.

Rarer anaemias such as DBA and pyruvate kinase deficiency are associated with variable rates of TIOL, depending on the underlying mutations. Sporadic blood transfusions for other production anaemia such as myelodysplastic syndrome (MDS) or multiple courses of myeloablative chemotherapy cause cumulative iron loading, which ultimately will need to be addressed with chelation.

Recently, the debate about optimal pretransfusion haemoglobin values in TDT and by implication other anaemias has been reignited because of reported improved survival in patients with pretransfusion values maintained at >100 g/L. Importantly, this analysis only contained patients with well-controlled iron overload (ferritin <800 µg/L). If iron overload is not well controlled, higher transfusion rates increase the risk of myocardial iron loading.

Consequences of Transfusional Iron Overload

Toxic consequences of TIOL vary with rate of loading, the duration of the iron overload and the underlying haematological disease in question. Broadly speaking, this reflects the distribution and concentration of storage iron derived from transfusion: these were first described in detail in TDT and remain the best understood. This is the same iron that is detected by MRI by T2, T2* techniques, so that the measurement of tissue iron concentration by MRI predicts iron-mediated toxicity, most usefully in liver and heart. As these MRI detectable iron stores are continuously turned over within cells, they generate free radicals and as they do so they cause membrane, organelle, and DNA damage

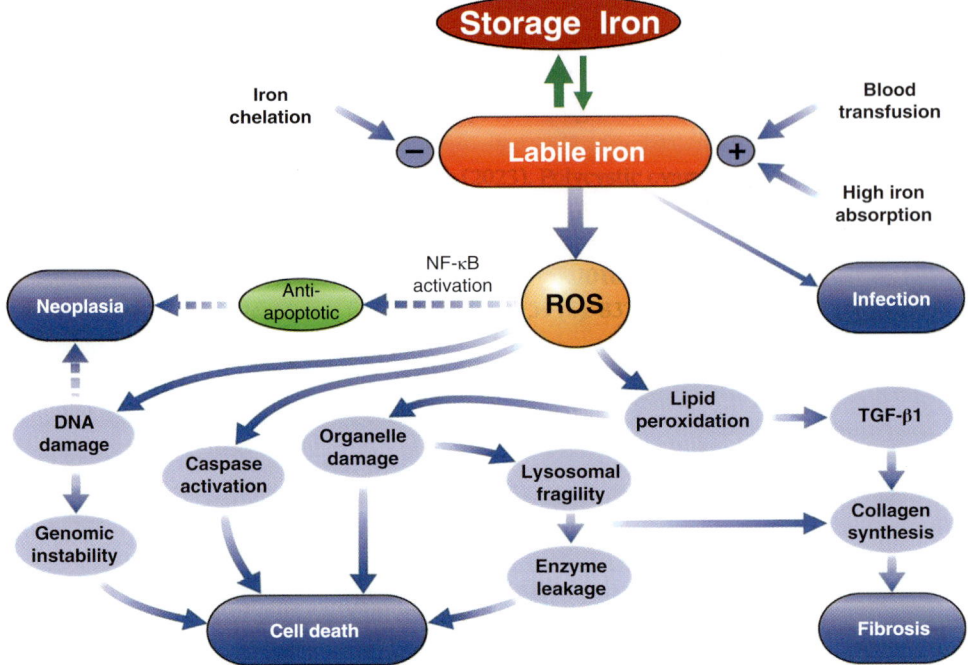

Figure 18.2 Pathological mechanisms of iron overload and toxicity. Iron excess leads to iron that is not liganded to naturally occurring molecules such as transferrin or ferritin and generates a variety of reactive oxygen species (ROS), most notably hydroxyl radicals. Labile plasma iron accumulates in cells, especially of the liver, endocrine tissues and myocardium. ROS increase lipid peroxidation and organelle damage, leading to cell death and fibrogenesis mediated by transforming growth factor, TGF β1 (Porter, 2005). ROS damage DNA, risking genomic instability, mutagenesis and cell death or neoplasia (Zuo et al., 2009). Paradoxically, ROS may also have anti-apoptotic effects by activating NF-kB (dashed lines) (Aggarwal, 2004), which may contribute to myelodysplastic transformation and to iron-mediated neoplasia such as hepatoma.

(Figure 18.2). Mechanisms of cell death include necrosis, apoptosis and the recently described ferroptosis. Ferroptosis can be inhibited experimentally with agents such as erastin and clinically using iron chelators.

Prior to the development of effective chelation, the predominant cause of death from TIOL was siderotic cardiomyopathy so that few patients with TDT lived into the third decade. Since the use of timely and effective chelation, these complications are less common in patients who adhere to daily treatment (see Chapter 26). Morbidity from TIOL still may include hypogonadotropic hypogonadism due to iron deposition in the anterior pituitary, with growth failure and later failure of puberty and fertility. Failure of this system contributes to the high rate of osteoporosis in these patients. Other endocrine glands commonly affected are thyroid, parathyroid and endocrine pancreatic function resulting in diabetes mellitus. In patients reaching their fifth decade and beyond, cirrhosis and hepatocellular carcinoma are increasingly seen. These patients require regular screening at least yearly for all these complications of iron overload.

Prevention of Transfusional Iron Overload

Prevention of TIOL depends on implementation of measures to reduce the need for transfusion. This includes use of alternative treatment strategies such as hydroxycarbamide for SCD, which raises HbF levels and reduces transfusion requirements.

Joint decision-making at the start of long-term transfusion programmes, such as in MDS, may improve tolerance to anaemia and enable longer intervals between transfusions. Early assessment, management and patient support with chelation therapy are paramount in reducing the clinical complications of TIOL.

Bibliography

Aggarwal BB. (2004). Nuclear factor-kappaB: the enemy within. *Cancer Cell* 6 (3): 203–208. doi: https://doi.org/10.1016/j.ccr.2004.09.003

Dixon, S., Lemberg, K.M., Lamprecht, M.R. et al. (2012). Ferroptosis: an iron-dependent form of nonapoptotic cell death. *Nature Chem Biol* 149 (5): 1060–1072.

Garbowski, M.W., Evans, P., Vlachodimitropoulou, E. et al. (2017). Residual erythropoiesis protects against myocardial hemosiderosis in transfusion-dependent thalassemia by lowering labile plasma iron via transient generation of apotransferrin. *Haematologica* https://doi.org/10.3324/haematol.2017.170605 102 (10): 1640–1649.

Musallam, K., Barella, S., Origa, R. et al. (2024). Pretransfusion hemoglobin level and mortality in adults with transfusion-dependent β-thalassemia. *Blood* 143 (10): 930–932.

Porter, J.B. and Garbowski, M. (2014). The pathophysiology of transfusional iron overload. *Hematol Oncol Clin North Am* 28 (4): 683–701, vi. doi: https://doi.org/10.1016/j.hoc.2014.04.003.

Porter JB and Garbowski M. A*merican Society of Hematology (*ASH) Educational Programme (2013). Consequences and management of iron overload in sickle cell disease. *Hematology Am Soc Hematol Educ Program* 2013 447-56 (https://doi.org/10.1182/asheducation-2013.1.447)

Shah, F., Porter, J., Sadasivam, N. et al. (2022). Guidelines for the monitoring and management of iron overload in patients with haemoglobinopathies and rare anaemias. *Br J Haematol* 196 (2): 336–350.

Vlachaki, E. and Venou, T.M. (2024). Iron overload: the achilles heel of β-thalassemia. *Transfus Clin Biol* 31 (3): 167–173.

Zuo, Y., Xiang, B., Yang, J. et al. (2009). Oxidative modification of caspase-9 facilitates its activation via disulfide-mediated interaction with Apaf-1. *Cell Res* 19: 449–457. https://doi.org/10.1038/cr.2009.19.

19

Haemochromatosis

Graca Porto

Hematology Serviço de Imuno-hemoterapia, CHUdSA-Centro Hospitalar Universitário de Santo António, Porto, Portugal

Introduction

Haemochromatosis (HC) is a unique clinical-pathological condition of genetic origin. It is the most common inherited condition of iron overload. It results from uncontrolled intestinal absorption of iron, leading to its high concentration in the blood with progressive accumulation in tissues, potentially resulting in disabling and/or life-threatening complications such as arthritis, diabetes, liver cirrhosis and hepatocellular carcinoma. The clinical-pathological hallmarks of HC are increased transferrin saturation (TSAT) and iron overload in the liver, but not in the spleen. The liver iron overload involves predominantly periportal hepatocytes with iron-spared Kupffer cells. The absence of anaemia or reticulocytosis distinguishes, by definition, HC from other iron loading anaemia or chronic haemolytic disorders that may present with similar phenotypes.

Pathogenesis

The pathogenic basis of HC is hepcidin deficiency, due to mutations in genes involved in the hepcidin-signalling pathway. Hepcidin is a small peptide hormone produced by the liver that negatively controls circulating iron levels through interaction with ferroportin, the only known cellular iron exporter in humans. By blocking ferroportin export capacity, hepcidin inhibits the absorption of dietary iron and iron release by spleen macrophages involved in iron recycling from senescent erythrocytes. As illustrated in Figure 19.1, hepcidin regulation by iron is complex, involving numerous players whose alterations can compromise hormone synthesis or function. Molecular defects causing hepcidin deficiency will result in uncontrolled intestinal iron absorption, with progressive iron accumulation in tissues.

By far the most common genetic alteration in HC is homozygosity for the p.Cys282Tyr (p.C282Y) variant in the *HFE* gene, defining the *HFE*-related HC. Rare forms of HC may be

Iron in Clinical Practice, First Edition. Edited by Sue Pavord and Noemi Roy.
© 2025 John Wiley & Sons Ltd. Published 2025 by John Wiley & Sons Ltd.
Companion website: www.wiley.com/go/medicine5e

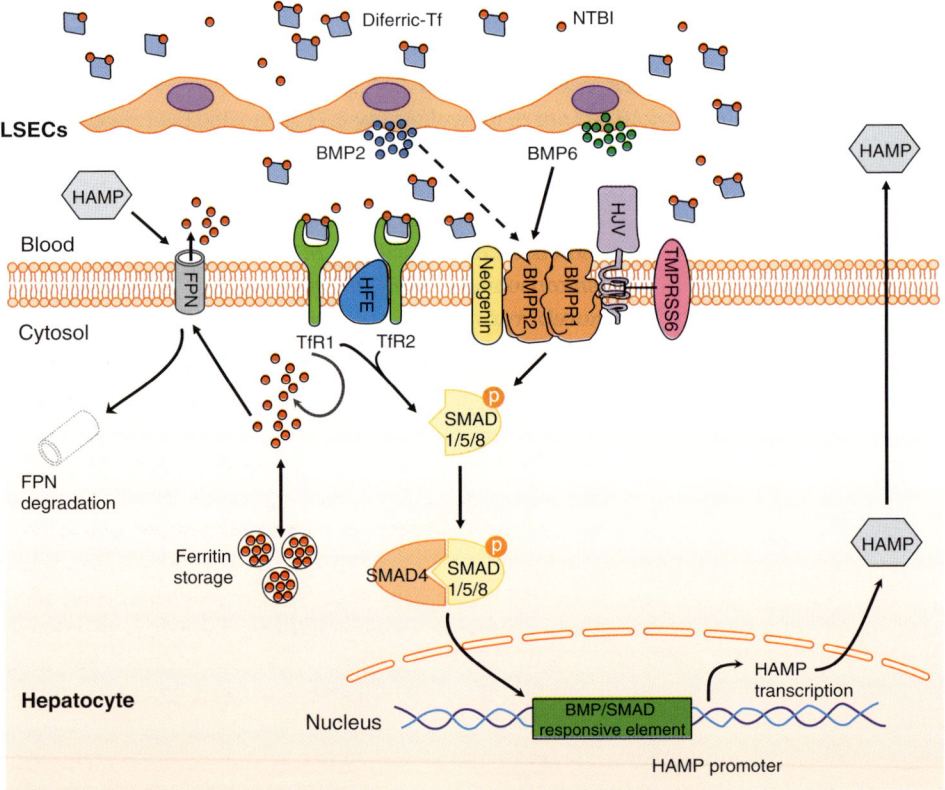

Figure 19.1 Hepcidin regulation by iron in hepatocytes. Increase in transferrin saturation induces hepcidin transcription via the BMP/SMAD signalling pathway. Diferric transferrin binds to TfR2, whilst BMP6 and BMP2 secreted by liver sinusoidal endothelial cells (LSECs) bind to BMP receptors on hepatocytes. These events trigger phosphorylation of regulatory SMAD1/5/8, recruitment of SMAD4 and translocation of the SMAD complex to the nucleus for activating hepcidin transcription upon binding to BMP/SMAD-responsive element in the *HAMP* promoter. BMPs can be trapped by ERFE (erythroferrone, a hormone produced by bone marrow erythroblasts), leading to inappropriate hepcidin inhibition in iron loading anaemias. Efficient iron signalling requires the BMP coreceptor HJV and the protein HFE and is negatively regulated by the transmembrane serine protease matriptase-2 (TMPRSS6). The complex molecular pathogenesis of HC reflects the numerous proteins involved in regulation of the hepcidin–ferroportin axis. *Source:* Adapted from Girelli et al. (2022).

caused by compound heterozygosity of the p.Cys282Tyr variant with other rare *HFE* pathogenic mutations or by homozygosity for pathogenic variants in other genes involved in hepcidin signalling or function, globally classified as non-HFE-related HC. A summary description of HC-associated genes, mode of transmission, geographical distribution and particular clinical features is presented in Table 19.1.

Frequency and Penetrance of *HFE*-Related Haemochromatosis

The p.Cys282Tyr variant is found at high frequencies in populations of European ancestry. It is particularly common in Northern Europe, namely in Ireland, where it reaches frequencies higher than 11%, meaning a probability of homozygosity higher than 1%

Table 19.1   Haemochromatosis (HC) classification, related genes, mode of transmission, geographical distribution and particular clinical features.

HC type	Gene	Mode of transmission	Geographical distribution	Clinical features
HFE-related	**HFE (p.Cys282Tyr)**	AR	Highest prevalence in Northern Europe	Adult onset; presents earlier and more severely in males; highly variable clinical expression, with predominant liver damage and arthritis
	HFE (non-p.Cys282Tyr)	AR		
Non-HFE-related	**HJV**	AR	Highest prevalence in Southern Asia	Juvenile: earlier onset (e.g.<30 years old); similar severity in both sexes; prevalent cardiac and endocrine involvement
	HAMP	AR	Several populations	
	TFR2	AR	Most frequent amongst non-Finnish European populations	Very rare (look for parental consanguinity); clinically similar to HFE-related, with an earlier onset
	SLC40A1[a]	AD	Several populations	Very rare; in general, clinically similar to *HFE*-related, but more severe/early-onset forms are reported

[a] *SLC40A1*-related HC refers to the very rare forms of HC due to variants leading to ferroportin resistance to hepcidin or impairing ferroportin stability or ability to export, which may result in conditions phenotypically and biochemically indistinguishable from hepcidin-deficient HC. This should be distinguished from the more common ferroportin disease, due to loss-of-function *SLC40A1* mutations characterised by distinctive clinical, biochemical and pathological features, which do not fit the definition of HC. AR, autosomal recessive. Adapted from Girelli et al. 2022.

(Figure 19.2). In spite of its high frequency, the clinical penetrance of *HFE*-related HC is relatively low in the general population, as revised from published data from a variety of empirical sources. In a recent large-scale study on community volunteers from the UK Biobank, it was shown that the cumulative incidence at 80 years for liver disease in the population of p.Cys282Tyr homozygotes was 20.3% versus 8.3% in the control population without *HFE* variants, and for liver fibrosis or cirrhosis, it was 7.7% versus 1.3%. These figures highlight the importance of enhancing case detection at early stages, before the development of liver cirrhosis, the well-established major factor impacting on the risk of liver cancer and life expectancy in HC patients.

Diagnosis

HC case detection requires a high degree of awareness and suspicion. Signs and symptoms are highly non-specific, the clinical manifestations resulting from impairments of the affected organs, namely, arthralgias, chronic fatigue, altered liver function tests, diabetes or

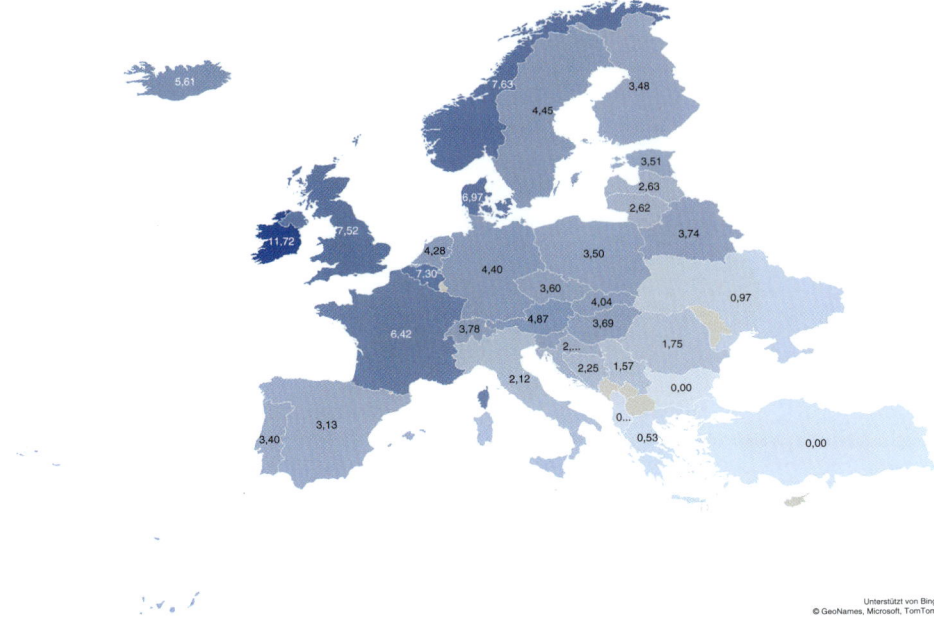

Figure 19.2 Prevalence of the p.C282Y risk allele for haemochromatosis in Europe. Note that allele frequency is subject to significant variation in specific geographical regions. One example for such variation is Portugal, where the risk allele prevalence is 5.8% in the North as compared to 0.9% in the South. *Source:* Adapted from European Association for the Study of the Liver (2022).

sexual dysfunction. The progressive iron accumulation is typically silent, those clinical manifestations generally occurring after the age of 40 years, predominantly in males. Women usually present later due to regular blood loss through menstruation/pregnancy. Nevertheless, the biochemical expression of the disease may be detected much earlier, during the preclinical stage. It consists of a sustained and unexplained abnormally high TSAT (more commonly >60% in males and >50% in females) and high serum ferritin, reflecting the increased iron stores. Ferritin alone, however, is not a predictor of HC, since it is highly non-specific and commonly found associated with other conditions such as chronic inflammation, excess alcohol intake or other chronic liver disorders. In Caucasians, a confirmed and unexplained high TSAT is a criterion to recommend a first-level *HFE* genetic test to search for p.Cys282Tyr homozygosity. *HFE* genotyping is also recommended as a predictive genetic test in all adult first degree relatives of confirmed p.Cys282Tyr homozygous patients, with proper counselling. However as mentioned before, p.Cys282Tyr homozygosity alone is not sufficient to make the diagnosis of HC. A formal diagnosis of HC implies the demonstration of liver iron overload, either indirectly by the inappropriately high serum ferritin or directly by measuring liver iron concentration with magnetic resonance imaging (MRI), or, more rarely, liver biopsy. Currently, efforts are being made amongst experts in the field to define reproducible cutoff levels of iron overload as assessed by MRI in an attempt to better define criteria of expressing HC.

In suspected cases with demonstrated severe liver iron overload and a negative first-level *HFE* test (i.e. not *p.Cys282Tyr* homozygous), a 'second-level' genetic test (or arguably first level in non-Caucasian or juvenile patients) should be considered to identify rarer variants in the *HFE* or in non-*HFE* genes known to be linked to hepcidin control, namely, *TFR2*, *HJV* or *HAMP*. Their molecular diagnosis is often complex, since variants in non-*HFE* genes are typically 'private', i.e. restricted to members of only one or a few families. In these cases, modern approaches based on next-generation sequencing (NGS), available at referral expertise centres, have greatly expanded the diagnostic possibilities of rare forms of HC.

Treatment and Prevention

The standard of care for HC remains therapeutic phlebotomies. These are performed intensively (weekly) in a first phase, intended to mobilise all the iron accumulated in the liver, followed by a second phase of regular phlebotomies (usually every 2–6 months) maintained to prevent iron re-accumulation. When performed at preclinical stages, regular phlebotomy effectively prevents the potentially fatal iron overload complications and provides normal life expectancy, supporting the importance of early diagnosis as the best preventive strategy in HC. In patients diagnosed at late stages, monitoring of iron overload complications in affected organs is required, particularly monitoring of hepatocellular carcinoma in patients who presented with liver fibrosis or cirrhosis. For reasons still not understood, HC arthropathy is the only complication that cannot be effectively treated by iron depletion therapy. Understanding HC arthropathy is presently one of the major unmet needs in HC research.

Bibliography

European Association for the Study of the Liver (2022). EASL clinical practice guidelines on haemochromatosis. *Journal of Hepatology* 77 (2): 479–502.

Girelli, D., Busti, F., Brissot, P. et al. (2022). Hemochromatosis classification: update and recommendations by the BIOIRON Society. *Blood* 139 (20): 3018–3029.

Grosse, S.D., Gurrin, L.C., Bertalli, N.A., and Allen, K.J. (2018). Clinical penetrance in hereditary hemochromatosis: estimates of the cumulative incidence of severe liver disease among HFE C282Y homozygotes. *Genetics in Medicine* 20 (4): 383–389.

Lucas, M.R., Atkins, J.L., Pilling, L.C. et al. (2024). *HFE* genotypes, haemochromatosis diagnosis and clinical outcomes at age 80 years: a prospective cohort study in the UK Biobank. *BMJ Open* 14 (3): e081926.

20

Ineffective Erythropoiesis

Noémi Roy

Department of Haematology, Oxford University Hospitals NHS Foundation Trust, Oxford, UK

Introduction

Erythropoiesis is the process by which red blood cells (RBCs) are produced from multipotent haemopoietic stem cells. This occurs in the bone marrow at a staggering rate of ~10^{11} new cells per day in steady state. These haematopoietic stem cells must mature through various erythroblast stages and terminally differentiate into enucleated biconcave discs, each filled with ~280 million haemoglobin molecules to transport oxygen to the tissues and carbon dioxide back to the lungs. This highly regulated system is dependent on both intrinsic and extrinsic factors to function normally. Any disruption of these factors can lead not only to a range of inherited or acquired anaemia but in certain cases also to iron overload.

Erythropoiesis

For the haematopoietic stem cells to develop down the erythroid lineage, a series of complex enhancers and transcription factors interact with each other and with epigenetic modifiers so that the erythroid 'programme' of genes is chosen and genes involved in the development of other haematological lineages are excluded. Some of these transcription factors, such as GATA-1, are well known, and the timing and levels of their expression determine whether a myeloid/erythroid progenitor develops down the red cell or megakaryocytic lineage. GATA-1 mutations can lead to a surprising number of different phenotypes, from amegakaryocytic thrombocytopenia, congenital dyserythropoietic anaemia, to porphyria.

Erythroblast development occurs in so-called islands with a central macrophage surrounded by erythroid precursors at different stages of maturation (Figure 20.1). These provide a specific microenvironment for proliferation and differentiation of the erythroid cells, including the provision of nutrients, survival signals and even possibly a role in the process of enucleation, with phagocytosis of the extruded nucleus as a final step.

(https://www.ncbi.nlm.nih.gov/pmc/articles/PMC3234703/)

Iron in Clinical Practice, First Edition. Edited by Sue Pavord and Noemi Roy.
© 2025 John Wiley & Sons Ltd. Published 2025 by John Wiley & Sons Ltd.
Companion website: www.wiley.com/go/medicine5e

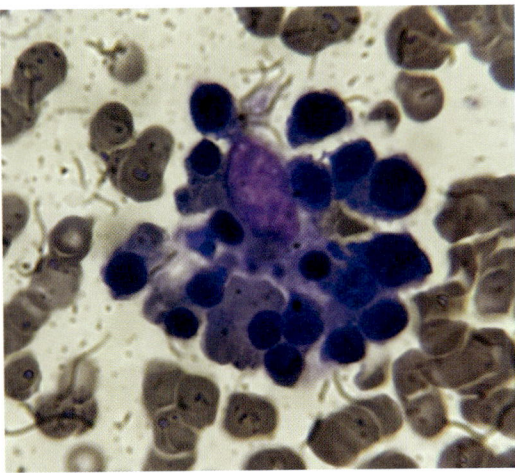

Figure 20.1 An erythroblastic island. X400 image of a normal bone marrow erythroblastic island.

The Role of Erythropoietin and Iron

While there are complex, highly tuned, interconnected processes that govern erythropoiesis, the pathway can nevertheless be divided into an initial 'EPO-dependent' phase, followed by an 'iron-dependent' phase. In the 'EPO-dependent' phase, erythropoietin (EPO) produced by oxygen-sensing cells in the kidneys travels to the bone marrow and binds EPO receptors on the surface of developing erythroblasts. Once bound, a signalling cascade is set in motion, the result of which is a 'survival signal' to the erythroblast. Importantly, there is always an excess of EPO receptor-bearing erythroblasts in steady state, such that some of these fail to receive the survival signal and naturally undergo apoptosis. While this may seem like a waste of resources, this redundancy, also termed 'ineffective erythropoiesis', has evolved as a way of ensuring a rapid response from the marrow in the context of sudden anaemia, such as would happen following a major bleeding episode. This would yield a rapid rise in EPO, and thus a rapid increase in erythroid precursors receiving the survival signal, and therefore a rapid increase in mature RBCs (Figure 20.2).

The iron-dependent half of the pathway is during terminal differentiation, at a time of maximal haemoglobin production. As seen in Chapter 2, iron that is either absorbed from the gut or recycled from senescent red cells, is transported by transferrin and binds transferrin receptors on the surface of developing erythroblasts, triggering clathrin-mediated endocytosis. Once the iron has been released from transferrin within the cell, it can be stored as ferritin or incorporated directly into haem.

The importance of matching alpha to beta globin is well known. Disturbance of this balance leads to thalassaemia, the world's most common genetic blood disorder. The normal haemoglobin molecule is made up of 2 alpha globin chains, 2 beta globin chains, 4 haem moieties and 4 iron atoms.

The incorporation of iron into protoporphyrin IX (PPIX) by the enzyme ferrochelatase (FECH) results in the formation of haem, which is then ready to be combined with globin to form haemoglobin. When this process is disrupted by genetic mutations, such as in sideroblastic anaemia, iron overload follows. These defects usually result from mutations in genes that code

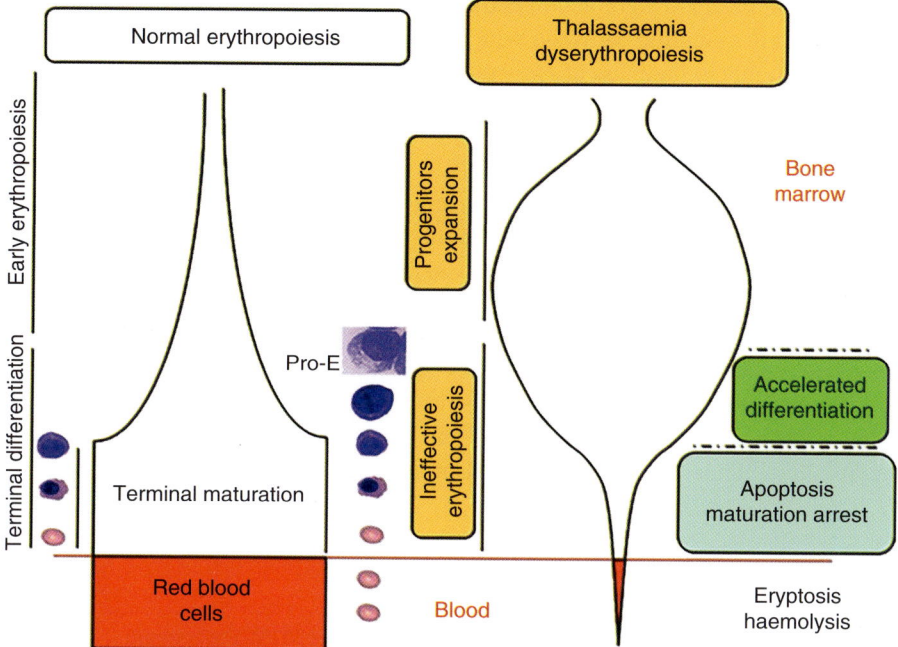

Figure 20.2 Ineffective erythropoiesis. A comparison of normal erythropoiesis with all types of ineffective erythropoiesis, such as in thalassaemia pictured here. *Source:* Ribeil et al. (2013)/John Wiley & Sons/CC BY 3.0.

for haem biosynthesis rather than directly for the incorporation of iron into haem, but their disruption leads to an accumulation of labile iron that fails to be utilised appropriately.

Ferrokinetic Studies

Ferrokinetic studies to track iron mobilisation, transport and cell uptake began in the 1960s, where subjects were injected with ^{59}Fe, a radioactive form of iron. Plasma iron turnover could be calculated by observing the clearance of ^{59}Fe from plasma. In steady state, this would be in the order of 4–8 mg/L/day. When found to be >8 mg/L/day in the absence of bleeding, this can indicate haemolysis or ineffective erythropoiesis (IE). These early studies were able to show the existence and extent of IE in a number of conditions, including thalassaemia. By definition, IE refers to those erythroblasts which undergo apoptosis while in the marrow and do not become a mature red cell.

Erythroferrone

As explained in Chapter 2, hepcidin is often referred to as the 'master regulator' of iron. However, the hormone erythroferrone (Erfe) controls the master controller itself. When Erfe levels are high, the effect of hepcidin is suppressed, irrespective of the body's iron status. One possible mechanism of action is that Erfe acts to trap the ligands (BMPs) that, when bound, activate signalling pathways which lead to hepcidin expression. Erfe levels in IE can be very high due to the mass of early erythroid precursors which are stimulated by high EPO levels in the context of anaemia. Thus a vicious cycle is triggered whereby low levels of mature RBCs lead to high EPO levels, increased survival of erythroid precursors which do not mature normally to functional RBCs, but suppressed hepcidin levels which continue to drive oral iron absorption despite excess body iron levels.

All forms of IE lead to iron overload through the suppression of hepcidin secondary to erythroferrone overproduction. Hepcidin levels are inappropriately reduced in all forms of IE, from thalassaemia and congenital dyserythropoietic anaemia to myelodysplastic syndrome. In the absence of hepcidin, ferroportin remains permanently 'open' and iron enters the bloodstream in an uncontrolled fashion. This iron, once it exceeds the storage capacity of transferrin and ferritin, becomes nontransferrin-bound iron (NTBI) and is taken up by hepatocytes, cardiac myocytes, pancreatic cells and the pituitary, eventually leading to cirrhosis, heart failure, diabetes and hypopituitarism, respectively.

Bibliography

Bou-Fakhredin, R., Rivella, S., Cappellini, M.D., and Taher, A.T. (2023). Pathogenic mechanisms in thalassemia I: ineffective erythropoiesis and hypercoagulability. *Hematol Oncol Clin North Am* 37 (2): 341–351.

Ribeil, J.A., Arlet, J.B., Dussiot, M. et al. (2013). Ineffective erythropoiesis in β -thalassemia. *Scientific World J* 2013: 394295. doi: 10.1155/2013/394295.

Shah, F.T., Porter, J.B., Sadasivam, N. et al. (2022). Guidelines for the monitoring and management of iron overload in patients with haemoglobinopathies and rare anaemias. *Br J Haematol* 196 (2): 336–350.

Shash, H. (2022). Non-transfusion-dependent thalassemia: a panoramic review. *Medicina (Kaunas)* 58 (10): 1496.

Tang, P. and Wang, H. (2023). Regulation of erythropoiesis: emerging concepts and therapeutic implications. *Hematology* 28 (1): 2250645.

Tomc, J. and Debeljak, N. (2021). Molecular insights into the oxygen-sensing pathway and erythropoietin expression regulation in erythropoiesis. *Int J Mol Sci* 22 (13): 7074.

Part 3b

Effects of Iron Overload on Body Organs

21

Iron Overload in the Heart

Malcolm Walker

Hatter Cardiovascular Institute, University College London Hospital, London, UK

Iron and the Heart

Iron is essential for the heart, not only as a major component of haemoglobin but also crucial in many enzymatic and metabolic processes that ensure normal myocyte function. Iron deficiency, even in the absence of anaemia, is associated with impaired cardiac performance (see Chapter 11). Iron overload can also be harmful, whether caused by dysregulated intestinal absorption as in haemochromatosis, excessive intake or due to repeated blood transfusion. Tissue accumulation of iron may occur in the heart and other organs. It is safely stored as ferritin and haemosiderin. However, if storage capacity is exceeded, free iron appears and leads to cell toxicity, impaired performance and, if not reversed, premature organ failure and death.

Cardiac Iron Regulation

Under normal, non-overloaded conditions iron enters myocardial cells via the ubiquitous mechanisms of transferrin-mediated endocytosis (TFR1) and divalent metal transporter (DMT1) receptors and removed through ferroportin. In the context of iron excess, once transferrin saturation capacity is exceeded, there is an increase in non-transferrin-bound iron (NTBI), which enters myocytes via L-type calcium channels (LTCC) (Figure 21.1).

Iron Overload

Although mutations in the haemochromatosis gene are very common in some parts of the world (1 in 150 to 1 in 300), homozygote *HFE* subjects with significant cardiac iron loading are uncommon, as the condition often presents with other organ dysfunction first, and venesection can be commenced prior to the development of clinically apparent myocardial

Iron in Clinical Practice, First Edition. Edited by Sue Pavord and Noemi Roy.
© 2025 John Wiley & Sons Ltd. Published 2025 by John Wiley & Sons Ltd.
Companion website: www.wiley.com/go/medicine5e

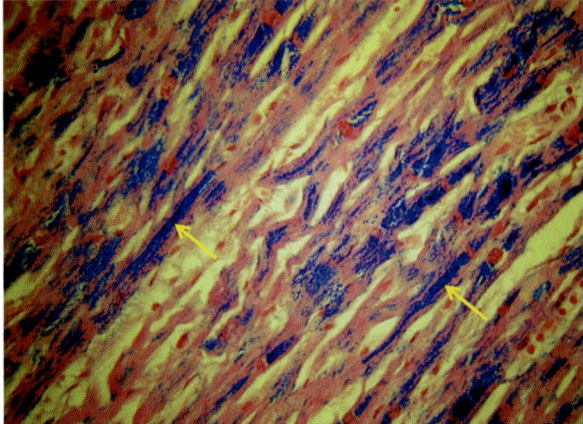

Figure 21.1 A myocardial biopsy, obtained with permissions, from a patient who died with severe cardiac iron overload. Myocytes contain blue stain (yellow arrows), illustrating the intra-myocytic deposition of iron, rather than deposited in the surrounding non-contractile tissue. *Source:* Kirk et al. (2016)/Elsevier/CC BY 4.0.

involvement (Chapter 19). Atrial fibrillation (AF) may be the exception, occurring early in some patients, prior to reduced pump function.

Secondary causes of iron overload occur with conditions requiring multiple transfusions. For this chapter, the experience gained from the thalassaemic syndromes will be used to draw conclusions for the other secondary iron overload conditions.

Worldwide there are approximately 60,000 births per year with severe thalassaemic syndromes, resulting in transfusion dependency for most of these patients. Once regular transfusion was demonstrated to be associated with survival beyond infancy, with improved growth, appearance and clinical function, the problem of iron overload due to transfused blood became apparent, since a normal adult's total body iron is exceeded 10-fold after just 4 years of monthly blood transfusion.

As the human has no endogenous mechanism to get rid of this excess iron, the chelators were introduced into clinical practice, initially desferrioxamine, which needs to be given parenterally, followed by the oral agents deferiprone and deferasirox (Chapter 26).

The future will include use of gene-based technologies, which have the prospect of achieving a cure by rendering patients free of transfusion dependency. We remain some distance from being able to deliver these therapies, particularly in the less developed nations. However, we will continue to rely on evidence-based therapies, which can achieve excellent results if applied early and assiduously.

Clinical Presentations and Their Management

Ventricular Dysfunction and Heart Failure

The heart, as other tissues, appears to be able to tolerate iron overload and exist for long periods in a state of high iron content with normal function, but under these circumstances, there exists a risk of sudden decompensation at times of increased demand or intercurrent illness. A young person with significant iron loading who suddenly presents with acute biventricular heart failure represents a true medical emergency, with a mortality risk of nearly 50%, even in experienced hospital environments. A more insidious presentation with a gradual development of increasing symptoms and signs of heart failure is now a more commonly encountered phenotype.

In both instances, intensification of chelation, with 24 hour, 7-day intravenous desferrioxamine plus an oral chelator such as deferasirox or deferiprone remains the mainstay of treatment, whilst meticulous attention to metabolic status, glucose control, consideration of adrenal insufficiency and control of precipitating infections or arrhythmia are also needed. Conventional heart failure treatments with renin-angiotensin-aldosterone system (RAAS) drugs are conducted, but often with limitations due to hypotension. Even without formal evidence to support RAAS drugs and newer agents, such as the SGLT2 inhibitors in these circumstances, it is wrong to withhold their use.

Stabilisation of acute decompensation often occurs quickly and should be followed by a period of chelation with combination treatments, usually desferrioxamine via the subcutaneous infusion route, 7 days per week plus an oral chelator, until function has normalised and cardiac iron reduced to a safer level (ideally an MRI T2* > 20 ms).

Arrhythmia

Arrhythmias are common in the iron-loaded population, particularly as they age, AF being the commonest issue encountered.

Although ventricular tachycardias (VT) used to be seen, these were accompanied by severe iron loading and, when present, invariably denoted a cardiomyopathy and immediate risk of sudden death. They respond acutely to parenteral desferrioxamine chelation, presumably due to immediate mopping up of labile, highly reactive iron in the blood. For this reason, the use of implantable defibrillators is rarely indicated in this subgroup of cardiomyopathy patients whose problem is caused by a removable toxin.

AF in a younger age group is usually a manifestation of significant iron overload and in those patients can be the precipitator of acute cardiac decompensation and needs to be reversed early, usually by urgent DC cardioversion. Paroxysmal AF is often encountered in the older patients, in up to 40% of patients with thalassaemia major over the age of 40 years. It can occur in the absence of current iron loading, although usually in patients who had a previous history of heart iron overload, up to 20 years previously.

The risk of venous thromboembolism is increased in this subpopulation, especially if they have had a splenectomy and anticoagulation should be considered in most patients.

Assessment of Cardiac Iron

Magnetic Resonance Imaging

Magnetic resonance imaging (MRI) using 1.5T machines is the only validated method to non-invasively detect tissue iron content. The MRI-based T2* parameter was the first method devised to assess myocardial iron, and its adoption into clinical practice led to a 70% reduction in cardiovascular mortality, by supporting the better use of the existing chelation therapies. It is still the only parameter that has been validated in human hearts against the physical quantitation of tissue iron content. The normal population T2* value is about 35 ms, and this is the target value set for most patients in the current era. A T2* over 20 ms confers a very low risk of cardiac complications, whereas a T2* <6 ms is associated with an approximate 50% risk of the development of heart failure within 12 months.

New, commercially available MRI sequences, enabling T2*, T2* mapping and T1 mapping, are becoming more widely available, with scanning times reduced to under 10 mins, drastically reducing costs. This means these advanced imaging techniques can be applied at scale, in countries where access to this technology was lacking.

Other Cardiac Tests

The electrocardiogram (ECG) is frequently, but non-specifically, abnormal in iron-overloaded patients, but some patients have a normal ECG, despite life-threatening levels of cardiac iron. ECG changes may not reverse when iron is removed.

Echocardiography is a widely available, safe, painless technique that provides instant, bedside cardiovascular assessment. The left and right ventricular ejection fraction (LVEF and RVEF) change late with iron overload although progressive reduction in LVEF or RVEF over time may alert clinicians to a developing problem, in this context, likely to be increasingly severe cardiac iron content. Newer modalities, such as tissue Doppler imaging (TDI) and global longitudinal strain measurements (GLS), have improved the sensitivity of echo assessment. Screening for the development of pulmonary hypertension, a particular issue with the non-transfusion-dependent thalassaemic populations can only practically be undertaken with echo but may need more detailed, invasive tests to fully characterise.

Cardiac biomarkers, such as NT-proBNP and troponin, have a very limited role in managing most patients with iron overload but are useful in acute decompensation.

Long-Term Management and Prevention

Successful management of cardiac complications depends on early detection and intervention (Table 21.1).

Prevention of accumulation of iron by regular surveillance screening, to inform the patients and their haematologists of their tissue iron loading, and the early introduction of effective chelation, tailored to the individual patient, have seen a progressive improvement in survival in transfusion-dependent thalassaemia patients, with a fall in cardiac complications (Figure 21.2). Part of this success has been the widespread adoption of combination chelation, often with the two oral preparations (deferiprone and deferasirox), which appears to result in improved long-term compliance. This leads to a reduction in cardiac iron content of approximately 23% over a 14-month period associated with an increase in the use of combination chelation from 19% to 37% of patients in a small study in India (Medina et al., 2022).

Table 21.1 Principles of successful management of cardiac complications.

Early assessment of iron loading.

Early introduction of chelation and the development of acceptable chelation regimes to the patient and their local healthcare system.

Surveillance to pick up cardiac involvement prior to overt heart decompensation.

Optimal treatment of cardiac complications, such as cardiomyopathy or atrial fibrillation.

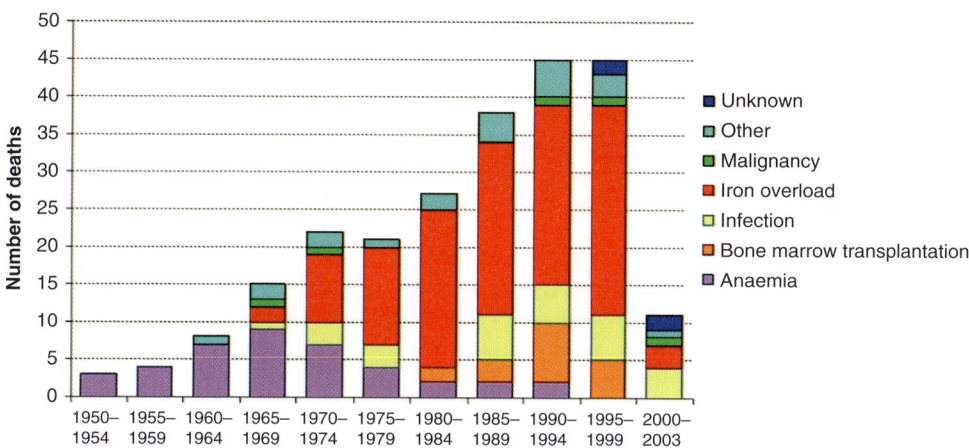

Figure 21.2 The UK thalassaemia cohort, showing deaths in intervals of 5 years. In 1999, the use of MRI, to obtain cardiac iron loading, became widely available to the doctors caring for these patients, who also had access to newer (oral) chelation to add to desferrioxamine. An improvement in survival followed with a 71% reduction in the annualised cardiac death rate (red portion of column). *Source:* Modell et al. (2008)/Elsevier/CC BY 2.0.

Prospective studies are needed to establish if regimes that include calcium channel inhibitors, such as amlodipine or verapamil, might further reduce iron loading, when used together with chelation. Other issues such as vitamin D status and control of conventional risk factors, such as hyperlipidaemia and diabetes, also provide the prospect of improved outcomes.

Chelation allied to careful surveillance with MRI has transformed a universally fatal disease of childhood into a condition that is now associated with the potential for a virtually normal lifespan. This is one of the more dramatic successes of medicine and pharmaceuticals.

Bibliography

Kirk, P., Sheppard, M., Carpenter, J.-P. et al. (2016). Post-mortem study of the association between cardiac iron and fibrosis in transfusion dependent anaemia. *J Cardiovasc Magn Reson* 19 (1): 36. https://doi.org/10.1186/s12968-017-0349-3.

Medina, K.M., Abdel-Gadir, A., Ganga, K. et al. (2022). Use of rapid cardiac magnetic resonance imaging to guide chelation therapy in patients with transfusion-dependent thalassaemia in India: UMIMI study. *Eur Heart J Qual Care & Clin Outcomes* 8 (3): 289–297. https://doi.org/10.1093/ehjqcco/qcab089.

Modell, B., Khan, M., Darlison, M. et al. (2008). Improved survival of thalassaemia major in the UK and relation to T2* cardiovascular magnetic resonance. *J Cardiovasc Magn Reson* 10 (1): 42. https://doi.org/10.1186/1532-429X-10-42.

22

Iron Overload and the Liver

Emma Saunsbury and Jeremy Cobbold

Department of Gastroenterology and Hepatology, Oxford University Hospitals NHS Foundation Trust, Oxford, UK

Introduction

Iron overload disorders result in increased total body iron stores and subsequent end-organ damage. As outlined in Chapters 18 and 19, iron can accumulate in the liver in a variety of congenital and acquired conditions, resulting in a spectrum of liver damage from minimal effects to liver fibrosis, cirrhosis and hepatocellular carcinoma (HCC).

Histological Patterns of Hepatic Iron Overload

The presence of granular iron in the liver is termed haemosiderosis, which can be stained for histologically with the Perls' Prussian blue stain. A normal liver does not show the presence of iron staining; therefore, any positive staining requires interpretation by a pathologist (Figure 22.1). Two main histological patterns of iron accumulation have been described. Primary iron overload predominantly involves parenchymal accumulation in hepatocytes and bile duct epithelium. Various grading systems exist to guide the subjective quantification of parenchymal iron. Scheuer's grading ranges from minimal (Grade 1) to diffuse accumulation that involves the entire lobule and obliterates the typical gradient (Grade 4). In contrast, secondary iron overload is seen mainly as accumulation in Kupffer cells, portal macrophages and endothelial cells.

Pathophysiology of Hepatic Damage Secondary to Iron Overload

The liver plays a central role in iron homeostasis. It has three key functions in regulating systemic iron concentrations: (i) it represents the main site for the production of proteins that maintain systemic iron balance, (ii) it is a storage site for excess iron and

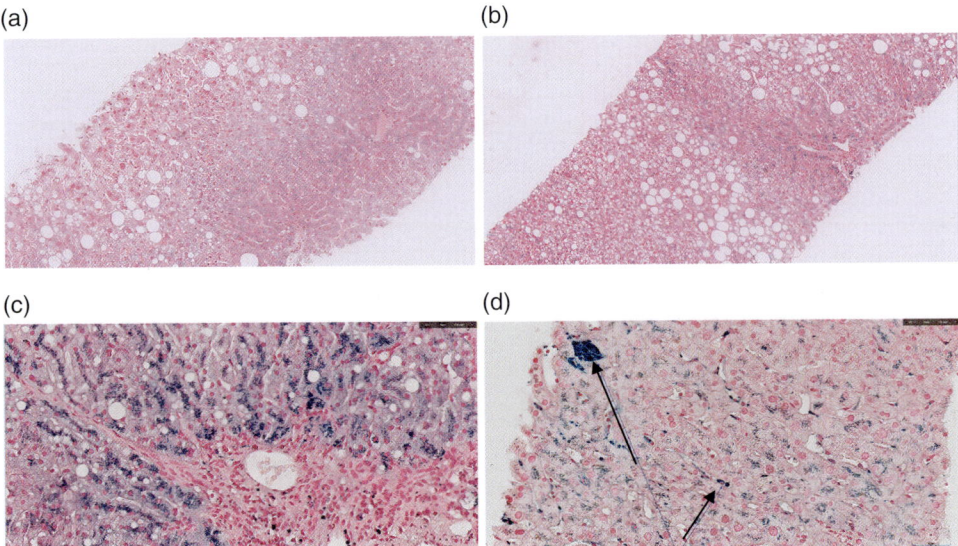

Figure 22.1 Patterns of hepatic iron accumulation, with Perls' Prussian blue staining to highlight haemosiderin granules in blue. (a) Grade 1 siderosis (in steatotic liver disease) (×200), (b) Grade 2 siderosis (in steatotic liver disease) (×200), (c) Grade 4 siderosis secondary to hereditary haemochromatosis, (d) secondary haemosiderosis secondary to blood transfusions, with iron in macrophages (arrows) as well as hepatocytes (×400). *Source:* Courtesy of Eve Fryer, Oxford University Hospitals NHS FT.

(iii) it mobilises stored iron back into the circulation to meet metabolic requirements. Hepcidin is the main iron-regulating protein produced by the liver, which inhibits intestinal iron absorption by binding to and degrading ferroportin (a cellular iron exporter located in the plasma membrane of intestinal enterocytes and macrophages) (see Chapter 2).

The principal mechanism of iron uptake in the liver is via transferrin, a protein which binds to iron resulting in a transferrin–iron complex. This is subsequently internalised into cells via receptor-mediated endocytosis. However, in severe cases of overload, iron levels will exceed the capacity of transferrin, meaning that labile nontransferrin-bound iron (NTBI) must be taken up by hepatocytes. As free intracellular iron is toxic, the majority of iron is stored in hepatocytes and Kupffer cells as ferritin, which can then be mobilized from the liver during times of high systemic demand of iron.

The liver increases its rates of iron storage in response to pathological systemic iron overload in order to protect other organs (e.g. the heart and pancreas) from iron-induced cellular damage. However, when its iron storage capacity is exceeded, iron-driven toxicity develops secondary to oxidative stress. Iron accumulation catalyses the Fenton reaction, increasing the generation of reactive oxygen species (ROS) via the decomposition of hydrogen peroxide by ferrous ion. ROS inflict oxidative stress on hepatocytes and Kupffer cells, causing cell damage through damage to cellular components including DNA, protein and lipids, stimulating apoptosis and the secretion of proinflammatory cytokines. ROS directly and indirectly trigger the activation of hepatic stellate cells (HSCs), which proliferate and differentiate into myofibroblast-like cells, contributing to

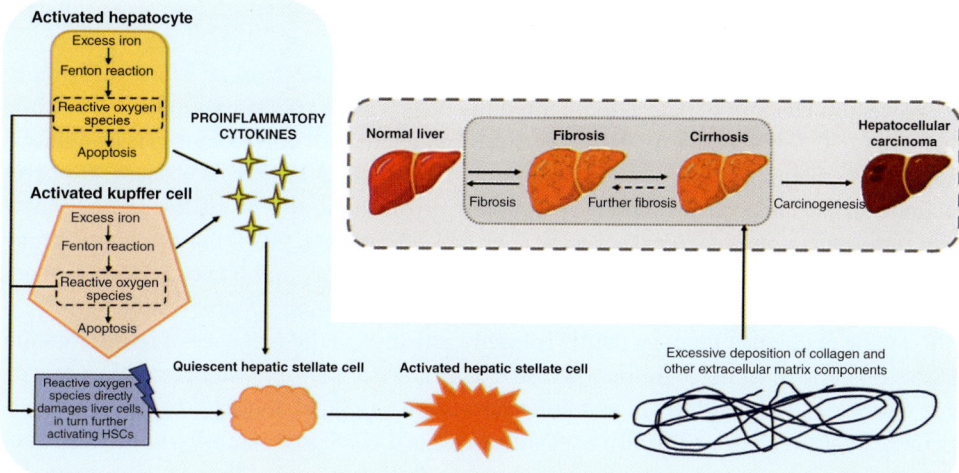

Figure 22.2   Intercellular pathways in fibrosis development.

the development of liver fibrosis through accelerated fibrinogenesis (i.e. excessive deposition of collagen and other extracellular matrix components within the hepatic parenchyma) (Figure 22.2).

Over time, the progressive liver fibrosis can lead to cirrhosis which can progress from a compensated, asymptomatic state to a decompensated state. Decompensated cirrhosis is characterised by the development of overt complications including ascites, jaundice, hepatic encephalopathy and/or variceal haemorrhage secondary to portal hypertension. Cirrhosis is also associated with an increased risk of HCC, as regenerating nodules in the cirrhotic liver develop atypical cells that progress toward dysplasia and neoplasia.

Conversely, iron accumulation can also occur in the liver secondary to chronic liver disease itself. The mechanism typically involves the reduction of hepcidin or impairment of its function. Disturbances in iron regulation are reported in diverse chronic liver diseases beyond haemochromatosis and are mostly associated with an adverse disease course.

Assessment of Hepatic Iron Overload

In order to avoid the development of such complications, accurate assessment methods are needed for detection, severity grading and treatment monitoring in patients with known or suspected iron overload.

Liver iron concentration (LIC) is linearly related to total body iron stores; therefore, its quantification is a reliable surrogate in assessing total body iron. A correlation has been demonstrated between serum ferritin concentration and LIC, particularly at higher values. However, as ferritin is an acute phase reactant, several confounding factors can exist, ranging from chronic alcohol excess and inflammation to metabolic syndrome and malignancy.

Ultrasound and computed tomography (CT) are commonly used, non-invasive imaging methods to evaluate the liver, but cannot quantify LIC.

Liver biopsy remains the reference method of assessing LIC. Normal LIC is <35 µmol/g of dry weight. Hepatic stellate cell functionality begins to be affected at >60 µmol/g, whilst cirrhosis typically develops at >250 µmol/g. The added benefit of liver biopsy is its ability to also provide diagnostic information about any underlying chronic liver disease. However, accurate assessment may be biased by sampling error, as the size of the liver biopsy specimen represents only 1/50,000th of total liver mass. Moreover, given the associated procedural complications (including haemorrhage, pneumothorax and bowel perforation) and cost involved, non-invasive investigations are preferred first-line where possible.

Magnetic resonance imaging (MRI) is highly sensitive to the presence of tissue iron and has become the first choice for non-invasive quantification of LIC where feasible. Over the past two decades, several MRI techniques have been validated and have been shown to be accurate over the entire clinically relevant ranges of LIC. Signal intensity ratio (SIR) compares the relative signal intensity of the liver to that of reference tissues not expected to exhibit iron overload (e.g. the paraspinal muscles) but therefore relies on the assumption that this reference tissue is normal. Alternatively, relaxometry can be utilised. Iron within liver accelerates the transverse relaxation of magnetisation from protons in water, leading to a concentration-dependent decay in signal intensity (e.g. "darkening" of tissue parenchyma on T2- and T2*-weighted imaging). This is sometimes alternatively reported as rates of signal decay (i.e. R2 or R2*), which are the reciprocal of T2 and T2*, respectively. T2* LIC estimation by MRI can be confounded by the presence of hepatic steatosis and fibrosis, nearby inhomogeneities and image noise. Patented R2 methods (FerriScan®) are more accurate than T2*methods but typically require off-site processing that involves additional cost, and therefore wider use is limited.

Transient elastography (FibroScan®) can be useful in non-invasively assessing liver stiffness, regardless of the degree of iron overload. Liver stiffness correlates with severity of liver fibrosis, but readings can be confounded by hepatic inflammation, hepatic congestion and body mass index amongst other factors, so it must be interpreted in the clinical context.

Bibliography

Batts, K.P. (2007). Iron overload syndromes and the liver. *Mod Pathol.* 20 (Suppl 1): S31–S39.

Chen, Q., Gao, M., Yang, H. et al. (2022). Serum ferritin levels are associated with advanced liver fibrosis in treatment-naive autoimmune hepatitis. *BMC Gastroenterol* 22: 23.

Cullis, J., Fitzsimons, E., Griffiths, W. et al. (2018). Investigation and management of a raised serum ferritin. *Br J Haematol* 181: 331–340.

Deugnier, Y. and Turlin, B. (2007). Pathology of hepatic iron overload. *World J Gastroenterol.* 13 (35): 4755–4760.

Di Marco, V., Bronte, F., Cabibi, D. et al. (2010). Noninvasive assessment of liver fibrosis in thalassaemia major patients by transient elastography (TE) - lack of interference by iron deposition. *Br J Haematol* 148 (3): 476–479.

Fernandez, M., Lokan, J., Leung, C. et al. (2022). A critical evaluation of the role of iron overload in fatty liver disease. *J Gastroenterol Hepatol.* 37 (10): 1873–1883.

Friedman, S.L. (2008). Mechanisms of hepatic fibrogenesis. *Gastroenterology.* 134 (6): 1655–1669.

Mehta, K.J., Farnaud, S.J., and Sharp, P.A. (2019). Iron and liver fibrosis: mechanistic and clinical aspects. *World J Gastroenterol.* 25 (5): 521–538.

Ramakrishna, G., Rastogi, A., Trehanpati, N. et al. (2013). From cirrhosis to hepatocellular carcinoma: new molecular insights on inflammation and cellular senescence. *Liver Cancer* 2 (3–4): 367–383.

Reeder, S.B., Yokoo, T., França, M. et al. (2023). Quantification of liver iron overload with MRI: review and guidelines from the ESGAR and SAR. *Radiology* 307 (1): e221856.

Zoller, H., Schaefer, B., and Vanclooster, A. (2022). EASL clinical practice guidelines on haemochromatosis. *J Hepatol* 77 (2): 479–502.

23

Impact of Iron Overload on the Endocrine System

Amy Morrison and Miles Levy

Department of Diabetes & Endocrinology, University Hospitals of Leicester NHS Trust, Leicester, UK

Introduction

In states of iron overload, endocrine organs are at a risk of damage due to iron deposition, with significant implications for hormone production. The most commonly affected endocrine organs are the pituitary gland and the pancreas, but effects are seen across multiple endocrine axes and should be assessed clinically.

Diabetes Mellitus

Diabetes mellitus, a dysregulation in glucose metabolism, is a recognised consequence of both direct iron deposition in pancreatic tissue and insulin resistance secondary to iron overload.

Pancreatic iron deposition, with resulting insulin deficiency and diabetes, is seen in around 50% of individuals with inherited haemochromatosis. It occurs in approximately 20–30% of adults with thalassaemia major and other severe transfusion-dependent anaemia who are poorly chelated.

Abnormal glucose regulation occurs as a result of reduced insulin sensitivity in the liver and adipocytes, increased hepatic glucose production and altered adipocyte fat metabolism, in addition to reduced insulin secretion. Pathways that influence glycaemia in a state of iron overload are depicted in Figure 23.1. Dysregulation in these endocrine pathways results in features of the metabolic syndrome, which may present clinically as type 2 diabetes or two or more of, elevated fasting glucose levels, elevated triglycerides, low HDL cholesterol, fatty liver, arterial hypertension and overweight/obesity. The concept of metabolic hyperferritinaemia traditionally requires a diagnosis of elevated ferritin levels (>300 ng/mL in men or >200 ng/mL in females) and evidence of fatty liver on biopsy

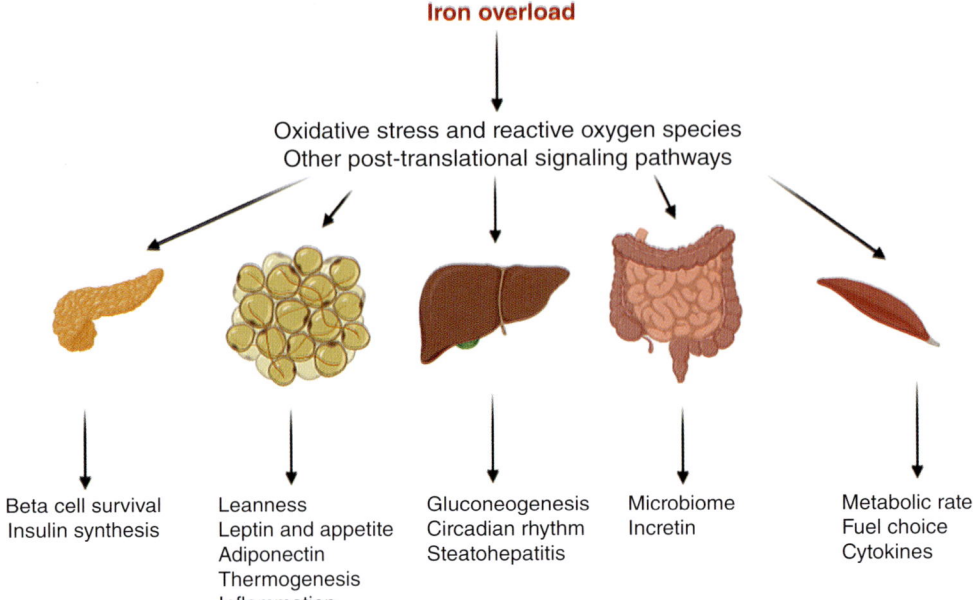

Figure 23.1   The multiple organs involved in the pathogenesis of diabetes in a state of iron overload. Pancreatic insulin secretion, metabolic parameters in adipocytes, hepatic glucose production and fat deposition, gastrointestinal microbiome and hormone release, in addition to inflammation and utilisation of substrate in skeletal muscle, determine predisposition to diabetes development in states of iron overload. *Source:* Adapted from Harrison et al. (2023).

imaging or non-invasive biomarkers. More recently these wider features of the metabolic syndrome have been identified to form part of this diagnostic algorithm.

Annual oral glucose tolerance test is a recommended screening tool for diabetes in all patients with transfusion-dependent thalassaemia and other transfused rare inherited anaemia. The standard diagnostic tool to assess for the presence of diabetes, glycated haemoglobin (HbA1c), is unreliable in the presence of haemoglobinopathies. A reduction in iron load, such as intensification of chelation therapy, is associated with a reduced incidence of diabetes.

Reproductive Endocrinology

Pituitary hormone production can be impaired by iron deposition. Hypogonadism is the most common effect of pituitary dysfunction associated with iron overload, due to iron deposition in pituitary gonadotroph cells, and an iron-induced oxidative stress. Resulting clinical presentations due to hypogonadism may include amenorrhoea, reduced libido and infertility. Non-elevated gonadotropin levels (luteinising hormone and follicle-stimulating hormone [LH and FSH]) in the context of low sex hormones (testosterone in men, oestradiol in women) identify underlying pituitary dysfunction, as opposed to primary gonadal

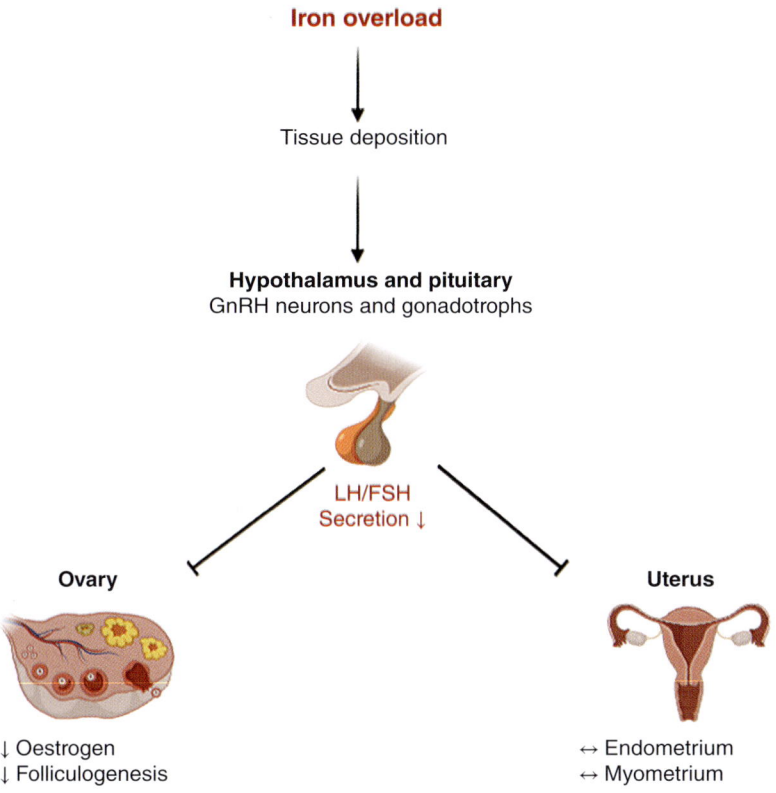

Figure 23.2 Proposed hypothalamicpituitary gonadal axis impairment in females secondary to acute iron overload (LH, luteinising hormone; FSH, follicle-stimulating hormone). *Source:* Adapted from Rossi et al. (2016).

involvement where LH and FSH are high. This can be followed up with confirmatory MRI imaging of the pituitary gland. Additionally, female rodent studies have identified iron overload toxicity at the level of the ovaries, with reduced oestrogen levels, reduced folliculogenesis, and increased ovarian reactive oxygen species. Ovarian, hypothalamic and pituitary dysfunction are all causes of impaired reproductive function seen in individuals with iron overload (Figure 23.2).

An additional area of reproductive endocrinology with links to iron overload is polycystic ovarian syndrome (PCOS), comprising a constitution of clinical and biochemical features including irregular menstrual periods, androgen excess and a polycystic appearance of the ovaries. PCOS is associated with elevated plasma ferritin, transferrin, iron and haemoglobin levels. PCOS is often associated with features of the metabolic syndrome including insulin resistance, type 2 diabetes, increased body weight gain and features that are apparent in states of iron overload such as in individuals with haemochromatosis. Metformin, the first-line medication initiated in the management of type 2 diabetes, is additionally often used as a therapeutic agent to improve insulin sensitivity in individuals with PCOS.

Growth and Bone Health

Iron overload can impact growth. Growth concerns are common in individuals with transfusion-dependent anaemia, resulting from a combination of chronic anaemia and iron overload. Growth hormone (GH) production from pituitary somatotrophs is another pathway at risk of dysfunction with iron overload. Before adulthood, short stature or failure of pubertal growth spurt should lead to the assessment of GH and insulin-like growth factor-1 levels (IGF-1 levels), followed by a GH stimulation test. This stimulation test is required to confirm GH deficiency prior to implementation of GH therapy, as low IGF-1 levels may be apparent in the frequent comorbidity of liver disease in these patients. This investigation is also indicated in adults if there is clinical concern or in the presence of another pituitary hormone deficiency.

Hypothyroidism may be an alternative cause for growth failure in children with iron overload. Iron overload may contribute to both primary and secondary hypothyroidism at all ages, and therefore checking thyroid-stimulating hormone (TSH) and free thyroxine levels can aid in the diagnosis and initiation of appropriate management with thyroxine replacement. Iron chelators can lead to improvement in hypothyroidism. With multiple conditions of iron overload leading to cardiac comorbidities, in which amiodarone therapy may be initiated, an awareness of the potential for amiodarone-induced thyroid dysfunction is also important in these patients.

GH plays a role in both the lengthening and density of bones. Bone mineral density is reduced in a state of iron overload, through an interplay of multiple contributory hormone pathways, which may lead to osteopenia or osteoporosis. GH deficiency impairs skeletal growth, due to decreased IGF-1-driven enhancement in bone remodelling and cartilage growth. Reduced androgen and oestrogen levels in coexisting hypogonadism result in increased bone resorption. In addition, the presence of hypothyroidism is associated with a reduction in bone turnover.

Increased bone resorption due to enhanced haematopoiesis can lead to suppression of parathyroid hormone production. Hypoparathyroidism can also rarely occur as a direct consequence of iron deposition in the parathyroid glands, resulting in symptomatic hypocalcaemia. Monitoring of calcium, phosphate and vitamin D levels and management with calcium and activated vitamin D supplementation is necessary in this scenario (Yang et al., 2020).

Adrenal Function

Adrenal insufficiency is a rare but potentially life-threatening complication of iron overload. It can occur at the level of the hypothalamus, pituitary or adrenal gland in states of iron excess. Clinical presentation resulting from steroid hormone deficiency includes symptomatic hypotension, low energy levels and weight loss. Assessment of the adrenal axis through baseline cortisol and adrenocorticotrophic hormone (ACTH), followed by ACTH stimulation testing, can be used to identify the need for steroid replacement.

Summary

An awareness of these potential areas of endocrine disruption in individuals with iron excess enables optimal screening of hormone deficiency and implementation of prompt, targeted management (Table 23.1).

Table 23.1 Assessment of endocrine dysfunction in individuals with iron overload.

Clinical presentation	Investigation	Management options
Hyperglycaemia		
Polyuria, polydipsia, weight loss	OGTT	Insulin Oral antidiabetic agents
Features of metabolic syndrome		
Hypertension, overweight/central obesity	Fasting glucose Lipid profile LFTs and liver imaging	Antidiabetic agents Lipid lowering therapy Weight loss interventions
Hypogonadism		
Amenorrhoea, low libido, infertility	LH, FSH Oestradiol, testosterone MRI pituitary	Hormone replacement therapy (HRT)
Growth		
Reduced height velocity	GH, IGF-1 GH Stimulation test TSH, T4	GH replacement Levothyroxine
Bone health concerns		
Low impact fractures	DEXA scan GH, IGF-1 TSH, T4 Oestradiol, testosterone	Bone protective agents including calcium and vitamin D GH Levothyroxine HRT
Hypoparathyroidism		
Symptomatic hypocalcaemia—tingling, numbness, muscle spasms	Calcium, phosphate Vitamin D PTH	Calcium and activated vitamin D
Adrenal Insufficiency		
Hypotension, fatigue, weight loss	U&Es ACTH, cortisol ACTH stimulation test	Replacement therapy – hydrocortisone (Fludrocortisone in primary adrenal failure)

OGTT, oral glucose tolerance test; LFT, liver function tests; LH, luteinising hormone; FSH, follicle-stimulating hormone; GH, growth hormone; IGF-1, insulin-like growth factor-1; TSH, thyroid stimulating hormone; T4, free thyroxine; PTH, parathyroid hormone; U&Es, urea and electrolytes; ACTH, adrenocorticotrophic hormone.

Bibliography

Harrison, A.V., Lorenzo, F.R., and McClain, D.A. (2023). Iron and the Pathophysiology of Diabetes. *Annu Rev Physiol* 85: 339–362. https://doi.org/10.1146/annurev-physiol-022522-102832.

Mathew, M., Sivaprakasam, S., Phy, J.L. et al. (2023). Polycystic ovary syndrome and iron overload: biochemical link and underlying mechanisms with potential novel therapeutic avenues. *Biosci Rep* 43 (1): BSR20212234. https://doi.org/10.1042/BSR20212234.

Pelusi, C., Gasparini, D.I., Bianchi, N., and Pasquali, R. (2016). Endocrine dysfunction in hereditary hemochromatosis. *J Endocrinol Invest* 39 (8): 837–847. https://doi.org/10.1007/s40618-016-0451-7.

Rossi, E.M., Marques, V.B. et al. (2016). Acute iron overload leads to hypothalamic-pituitary-gonadal axis abnormalities in female rats. *Toxicology Letters* 240 (1): 196–213.

Valenti, L., Corradini, E., Adams, L.A. *et al.* Consensus statement on the definition and classification of metabolic hyperferritinaemia. *Nat Rev Endocrinol* 19, 299–310 (2023). https://doi.org/10.1038/s41574-023-00807-6

Yang, W.P., Chang, H.H., Li, H.Y. et al. (2020). Iron overload associated endocrine dysfunction leading to lower bone mineral density in thalassemia major. *J Clin Endocrinol Metab* 105 (4): dgz309. https://doi.org/10.1210/clinem/dgz309.

24

Iron Overload and the Musculoskeletal System

Kassim Javaid

The Botnar Centre, Nuffield Orthopaedic Centre, Oxford, UK

Introduction

The effect of iron overload (IOL) on bone health is multifactorial. IOL has direct effects on osteoblast bone formation and osteoclastic bone resorption as well as indirect effects through hypogonadism, hypoparathyroidism, hypothyroidism, diabetes and chronic liver disease (Figure 24.1). There may be additional effects through hepcidin deficiency in haemochromatosis, thalassaemia, marrow expansion and sickle cell disease, such as bone infarction, as well as uncommon potential bone complications from iron chelation therapy. In general, chelation therapy improves bone health.

The primary effects of IOL on musculoskeletal health are an increased risk of osteoporosis, fragility fractures and osteoarthritis (OA).

Osteoporosis and Fracture Risk

In cohort studies, up to a third of adults with haemochromatosis have densitometric osteoporosis. The risk of hip fracture was significantly higher in homozygous *HFE* p.C282Y men but not in women or men with compound heterozygous variants. In some cohorts, younger adults do not present with complete fractures but more bone marrow oedema-like syndromes.

Iron toxicity and reactive oxidative stress increase osteoclast differentiation and resorbing activity. There is also increased RANKL mRNA production by iron-stimulated osteocytes. IOL reduces osteoblast proliferation and potential mineralisation by iron-binding phosphate to inhibit hydroxyapatite formation or by iron-inhibiting osteoblast tissue non-specific alkaline phosphatase, as well as calcium bioavailability by inhibiting vitamin D activation.

Iron in Clinical Practice, First Edition. Edited by Sue Pavord and Noemi Roy.
© 2025 John Wiley & Sons Ltd. Published 2025 by John Wiley & Sons Ltd.
Companion website: www.wiley.com/go/medicine5e

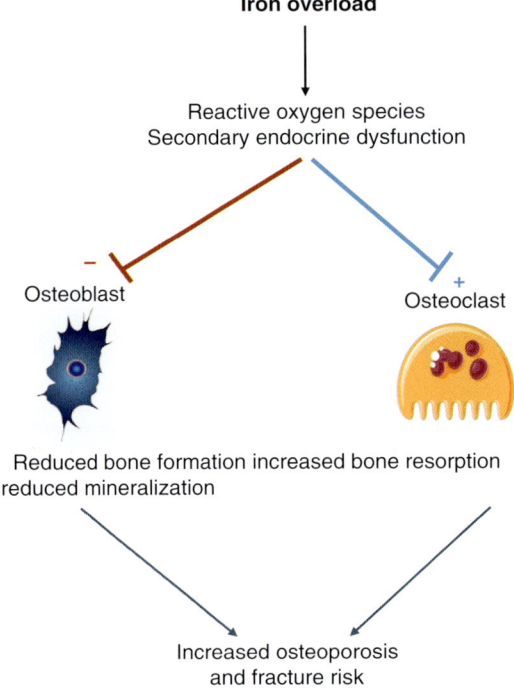

Iron overload

Reactive oxygen species
Secondary endocrine dysfunction

Osteoblast

Osteoclast

Reduced bone formation increased bone resorption
reduced mineralization

Increased osteoporosis
and fracture risk

Figure 24.1   Iron overload and bone health.

Assessment and management of bone health follows strategies for patients without IOL, with extra regard to excluding secondary causes from related endocrine dysfunction. The fracture risk assessment tool (FRAX), which estimates an individual's 10-year probability of incurring a hip or other major osteoporotic fracture, does not include IOL as one of the secondary causes of osteoporosis. Furthermore, it is not clear if all the fracture risk is captured by bone density. Options include selecting the rheumatoid arthritis input on FRAX as is recommended for type II diabetes, but this is not evidence based.

Whilst the mechanism of bone loss includes both increases in bone resorption and reduction in bone formation, current therapeutic strategies are similar for higher fracture risk patients without IOL and include calcium and vitamin D repletion and anti-osteoporosis medication.

Osteoarthritis

The OA caused by IOL is similar to generalised OA except for the predilection for the second and third metacarpophalangeal joints and large joints and other joints such as the ankle. Using the UK BioBank, the homozygous *HFE* p.C282Y variant is associated with a premature diagnosis of OA and hip and knee arthroplasty. The risk is more significant in males for both OA and hip/knee replacement compared with females, which may reflect disease severity and healthcare access. Further, arthroplasty risk was greater for homozygous males than for compound heterozygous or heterozygous men.

Calcium Pyrophosphate Deposition Disease

Calcium pyrophosphate deposition disease (CPPD) is another complication that affects 25% of patients with IOL. CPPD can present with severe attacks of inflammatory arthritis but may also become persistent with intermittent flare patterns that could be confused with seronegative inflammatory arthropathies. Moderate synovitis is typically found on ultrasound, more than would be expected with generalised OA. Whilst joint aspiration for pyrophosphate crystals is the gold standard, plain radiographs can demonstrate chondrocalcinosis in the knee, ankle and wrist. The characteristic radiographic findings are hook osteophytes in the second and third metacarpals (Figure 24.2), but this is not present in all patients.

Management of Iron Overload in the Joints

Joint pain can improve, be unchanged or worsen with iron removal. Timing of joint replacement surgery for moderate to severe pain is critical, balancing symptom severity with the expected timeline for revisions with expert orthopaedic review. Lifestyle advice, weight optimisation and general exercise, as well as specific muscle group targeted physical therapy strategies, may delay arthroplasty.

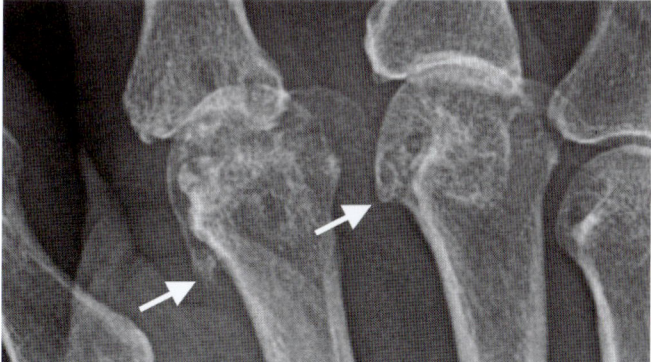

Figure 24.2 Metacarpal hook osteophytes in hereditary haemochromatosis. *Source:* ESIMR / http://preview.fluidmedia.com/UncoveringHandRadiograph/images/imagingfeatures/ Osteophyte2.jpg.

Bibliography

Banfield, L.R., Knapp, K.M., Pilling, L.C. et al. (2023). Hemochromatosis genetic variants and musculoskeletal outcomes: 11.5-year follow-up in the UK Biobank cohort study. *BMR Plus* 7: e10794.

Gregson, C.L., Armstrong, D.J., Bowden, J. et al. (2022). K clinical guideline for the prevention and treatment of osteoporosis. *Arch Osteoporos* 17: 58.

Mitton-fitzgerald, E., Gohr, C.M., Williams, C.M., and Rosenthal, A.K. (2022). Identification of common pathogenic pathways involved in hemochromatosis arthritis and calcium pyrophosphate deposition disease: a review. *Curr Rheumatol Rep* 24: 40–45.

Robin, F., Chappard, D., Leroyer, P. et al. (2023). Differences in bone microarchitecture between genetic and secondary iron-overload mouse models suggest a role for hepcidin deficiency in iron-related osteoporosis. *Faseb J* 37: e23245.

Von brackel, F. N. & Oheim, R. (2024). Iron and bones: effects of iron overload, deficiency and anemia treatments on bone. *JBMR Plus* 8: ziae064.

Part 3c

Assessment and Management of Iron Overload

25

Assessment of Iron Overload

Subarna Chakravorty

Department of Paediatric Haematology, King's College Hospital, London, UK

Introduction

Excess iron is toxic to organs but cannot be excreted by the human body by physiological means. Early detection of iron overload (IOL) is crucial in avoiding organ damage by allowing the timely initiation of iron chelation therapy.

Assessment of IOL can be undertaken by several means including history and clinical examination, biochemical testing of blood or tissue samples, or by radiological methods. All modalities of assessment are associated with pitfalls, and no investigation is necessarily adequate without an appropriate clinical context.

Awareness of Potential Causes

In many cases, particularly in those with repeated transfusions, the potential for IOL is not considered, and toxicity with cell death is allowed to continue, further exacerbating anaemia and leading to more transfusions. Awareness of the risk of IOL is essential to avoid this negative spiral of events. Potential causes of IOL are shown in Table 25.1.

Assessment of Transfusional Iron Overload

Transfusion-dependent anaemia leads to IOL, necessitating chelation therapy. Each unit of packed red blood cells contains 200–250 mg of iron, and after >10 transfusions, iron accumulation can cause toxicity. As IOL progresses, transferrin becomes fully saturated, leading to the formation of toxic nontransferrin-bound iron, free radicals, cell death, and fibrosis.

Table 25.1 Conditions that may lead to iron overload, through ineffective erythropoiesis and/or repeated transfusions.

Inherited

Transfusion-dependent thalassaemia (TDT)

Nontransfusion-dependent thalassaemia (NTDT)

Transfused sickle cell disease

Rare inherited anaemia–
Congenital sideroblastic anaemia, congenital dyserythropoietic anaemia, Diamond Blackfan anaemia

Red cell enzymopathies –
Pyruvate kinase deficiency, G6PD deficiency

Membranopathies –
Hereditary spherocytosis, hereditary elliptocytosis

Disorders in haem synthesis pathways

Acquired

Myelodysplastic syndrome

Aplastic anaemia

Red cell aplasia

Chronic myelofibrosis

Autoimmune haemolytic anaemia

Paroxysmal nocturnal haemoglobinuria

Systemic anticancer therapy

Bone marrow transplantation

Clinical history of transfusion duration, frequency, and volume is crucial for assessing iron accumulation. Rate of iron loading (ROIL) can be calculated using the following formula:

$$\text{Rate of iron loading: mg/kg/day} = \frac{\text{units of blood transfused} \times 200}{\text{Weight} \times \text{days over which blood was transfused}}$$

$$\text{Rate of iron loading: mg/kg/day} = \frac{\text{mL of blood transfused} \times 1.08}{\text{Weight} \times \text{days over which blood was transfused}}$$

Patients with an average ROIL between 0.3 and 0.5 mg/kg/day will typically need average chelator doses. However, those with a ROIL below 0.2 mg/kg/day or above 0.5 mg/kg/day will require dose adjustments accordingly.

Role of Serum Ferritin and Iron Studies in Assessing Iron Overload

Excess iron from transfusions or increased absorption is stored in the reticuloendothelial system via ferritin. In transfusion-dependent thalassaemia (TDT), serum ferritin levels can linearly reflect iron stores, especially if the iron load is not severe. For TDT patients with a history of transfusions for over 12 months, a serum ferritin level above 1000 ng/mL on two or three readings, one month apart, indicates the need for iron chelation therapy to prevent organ damage. Following initiation of chelation therapy, ferritin should be monitored every three months to adjust chelator dose. Chelation must be reduced or paused if ferritin drops below 300–500 ng/mL to avoid toxicity. In conditions like Diamond Blackfan anaemia or nontransfusion-dependent thalassaemia (NTDT), ferritin often underestimates iron levels; thus, radiological assessments and transfusion history are crucial for chelation decisions. If magnetic resonance imaging (MRI) is unavailable, serum ferritin above 800 ng/mL can guide NTDT chelation.

In genetic haemochromatosis, ferritin levels above 150–200 ng/mL in menstruating women and above 300 ng/mL in males or postmenopausal women may indicate IOL, warranting referral and management with chelation or phlebotomy to prevent organ damage, with the goal of reducing ferritin to below 300 ng/mL. MRI can further assess organ iron accumulation.

Serum iron varies diurnally and reflects a labile iron pool and is not a useful test to assess iron status. Transferrin-bound iron is a good measure of iron in the circulation and in IOL is significantly saturated to >60% of available transferrin molecules. This is often a good preliminary test to indicate underlying iron burden, so that further definitive investigations can be initiated. Total iron binding capacity of transferrin measured directly or indirectly (from serum iron and unsaturated iron binding capacity) is helpful in assessing the degree to which the transferrin is saturated in IOL.

Imaging in Iron Overload

MRI of the liver and heart using standardised protocols is currently the gold standard in assessing organ iron loading in transfusion-dependent anaemia. In 2001, Pennell and colleagues developed and validated the use of MRI T2* modality to assess cardiac IOL in TDT patients. The T2* values (in milliseconds) inversely correlate with iron loading of the heart, and prospective studies have helped establish clinical algorithms to predict likelihood of cardiac failure based on cardiac T2* measurements.

Before the advent of MRI, histological analysis of liver biopsy samples for iron quantification was used for assessing liver iron concentration (LIC). However, this has been mostly replaced by non-invasive MRI techniques. R2 relaxometry, specifically FerriScan®, is a widely available and FDA-approved technique for 1.5-T MRI scanners. This method has strong correlation with LIC and is widely used in clinics and research studies. It is often considered the gold standard due to its cross-site and cross-platform validation, as well as ongoing quality control and assurance measures. However, the technique requires a lengthy imaging time (~20 minutes), which often necessitates sedation for paediatric patients. The data processing is complex, involving centralised analysis, and the instruments must be calibrated beforehand. Additionally, a service fee per patient is charged for data analysis, on top of the MRI scan cost, limiting its widespread adoption.

R2* relaxometry is an alternative method with a linear correlation to LIC. There is no consensus on the ideal image acquisition method for this technique; many centres use custom sequences and postprocessing software with their own LIC calibration. R2* relaxometry is however a quick technique, requiring only one breath-hold, and can quantify LIC up to 20 mg/g dry weight using 1.5-T scanners. However, inaccuracies persist at high iron concentrations, and this is not the preferred modality when iron burden is high such as

Table 25.2 Clinical interpretation of liver and cardiac iron overload by MRI parameters.

Clinical interpretation of liver iron concentration by R2 relaxometry (FerriScan™ values)

LIC range	Clinical relevance
0.17–1.8 mg Fe/g dw	Normal range in nondisease patients in healthy population
3.2–7.0 mg Fe/g dw	Suggested optimal range of LIC for chelation therapy in transfusional iron loading
7.0–15.0 mg Fe/g dw	Increased risk of complications
>15.0 mg Fe/g dw	Greatly increased risk of cardiac disease and early death in patients with transfusional iron overload
	A follow-up FerriScan may be required every 6–12 months

Clinical interpretation of cardiac T2* values

T2* value	Clinical relevance
T2* > 20 ms	Cardiac iron deposition is not apparent
T2* 10–20 ms R2* 50–100/s	Some cardiac iron deposition has occurred, but there is little immediate risk of iron-induced cardiac decompensation
T2* < 10 ms R2* > 100/s	Significantly increased risk of iron-induced cardiac decompensation

that occurs in transfusional IOL. Table 25.2 highlights the clinical correlation of cardiac T2* and liver R2 relaxometry (FerriScan) measurements

Monitoring Requirements for At-risk Patients

The monitoring requirements for patients at risk of IOL are outlined in Table 25.3.

Table 25.3 Monitoring of individuals at risk of iron overload.

1) Yearly transfusional iron loading and blood volume calculation.
2) Ferritin measurement every 1–3 months for trend analysis.
3) Regular MRI surveillance for cardiac and liver iron in adults and children >8 years who can undergo scanning without sedation. For younger children with severe iron overload, MRI may require sedation.
4) Annual left-ventricular ejection fraction assessment from age 8 and arrhythmia evaluation for patients with palpitations.
5) Liver fibrosis screening in patients over 40 years and for hepatocellular carcinoma every 6 months in those with severe liver iron overload or previous hepatitis C.
6) Nontransfusion-dependent thalassaemia: Liver MRI if baseline ferritin is above 800 ng/mL and repeat as indicated.
7) Nontransfusion-dependent rare anaemia: Baseline liver and cardiac MRI if ferritin exceeds 1000 ng/mL.

Bibliography

Anderson, L.J., Holden, S., Davis, B. et al. (2001). Cardiovascular T2-star (T2*) magnetic resonance for the early diagnosis of myocardial iron overload. *Eur Heart J* 22 (23): 2171–2179.

Kowdley, K.V., Brown, K.E., Ahn, J., and Sundaram, V. (2019 Aug). ACG clinical guideline: hereditary hemochromatosis. *Am J Gastroenterol.* 114 (8): 1202–1218.

Shah, F.T., Porter, J.B., Sadasivam, N. et al. (2022). Guidelines for the monitoring and management of iron overload in patients with haemoglobinopathies and rare anaemias. *Br J Haem* 196 (2): 336–350.

Taher, A.T., Viprakasit, V., Musallam, K.M., and Cappellini, M.D. (2013). Treating iron overload in patients with non-transfusion-dependent thalassemia. *Am J Hematol.* 88 (5): 409–415.

26

Management of Iron Overload

Nandini Sadasivam

Department of Haematology, Manchester Royal Infirmary, Manchester, UK

Introduction

In the presence of anaemia and iron overload, iron chelation is the treatment of choice, whilst venesections are preferred in hereditary haemochromatosis where haemoglobin concentration is normal. The goal of iron chelation is to maintain a safe level of body iron, thus preventing iron deposition in body organs and the development of clinical complications.

Iron Chelation Therapy

There are currently three available iron chelating agents that may be used alone or in combination (Table 26.1). The chelators bind iron to form iron–chelate complexes, which are then excreted via the faecal or urinary route. The circulating active chelator controls and reduces direct tissue damage caused by the toxic nontransferrin-bound iron and only works whilst present in the circulation. Chelation reduces liver storage iron more quickly than from the heart and other tissues. Thus, heart iron values (when T2* is <20 ms) may lag behind that of the liver.

Once iron has accumulated, depending on the severity of iron loading, it can take several years to achieve an iron-neutral state as there is only a finite pool of chelatable iron at any one time.

Indications for Iron Chelation Therapy

People who require iron chelation include those with transfusion-dependent anaemia, for example, beta thalassaemia major, or other rare inherited anaemia such as Diamond Blackfan anaemia and sideroblastic anaemia (see Chapter 20), as well as people who

Iron in Clinical Practice, First Edition. Edited by Sue Pavord and Noemi Roy.
© 2025 John Wiley & Sons Ltd. Published 2025 by John Wiley & Sons Ltd.
Companion website: www.wiley.com/go/medicine5e

Table 26.1 Available chelation regimens.

Available Chelation Regimens
Desferrioxamine
Deferasirox
Deferiprone
Desferrioxamine and deferiprone
Desferrioxamine and deferasirox
Deferasirox and deferiprone

develop transfusion dependence later in life, for instance, with myelodysplastic syndrome. Some patients with ineffective erythropoiesis, such as those with congenital dyserythropoietic anaemia or nontransfusion-dependent thalassaemia, may suffer from nontransfusional iron overload and require chelation intermittently throughout life. In addition, individuals with inherited or acquired haemolytic anaemia may need iron chelation particularly if regular transfusions are given to maintain haemoglobin. Finally, bone marrow transplant patients may also require a period of chelation following their transplant if multiple transfusions have been administered.

Administration of Iron Chelation Therapy

Iron chelation can be challenging for some people (Table 26.2), particularly when faced with life pressures, such as is often seen with adolescents. Clinical teams need to be non-judgemental, responsive, and find a solution suited to the individual to improve adherence. When all outpatient-based treatments have failed in a patient with significant iron loading, attempts should be made for inpatient intensification of chelation.

Combination Chelation Therapy

Combination chelation therapy may be required in the following circumstances:

1) to increase the overall exposure to iron chelation when monotherapy at licensed doses is insufficient;
2) when monotherapy is limited by dose-dependent toxicity;
3) when compliance with monotherapy at the required frequency is inadequate; and
4) when simultaneous chelators have the potential to synergistically increase cellular iron removal rates.

   The decision about combination therapy is made together with the specialist multidisciplinary team and the patient (Table 26.3). All chelators work if taken at the correct doses and frequencies. One chelator option is not used throughout a patient's life. Chelators may need rotating or changing at different time points (Table 26.4). For example, appropriate

Table 26.2 Iron chelation regimens with monotherapy options.

	Route	Half life	Administrative challenges
Desferrioxamine	Subcutaneous or intravenous Infusion typically runs over 8–12 hours Given for 3–6 days a week	20–30 mins	Effective if taken in the right doses and frequency, but this is challenging for individuals in day-to-day life Adverse effects include: • Local skin reaction – addition of hydrocortisone to vials/devices can be helpful • Hypersensitivity may require a desensitisation program. • Infection with *Yersinia enterocolitica* requires discontinuation of Desferrioxamine until treated, whereas deferiprone or deferasirox can be continued • Desferrioxamine should also be stopped with *Klebsiella* infection or sepsis with other encapsulated bacteria
Deferasirox	Oral daily	12–16 hours	Preferred first--line option as it is oral administration and once daily Occasionally gastrointestinal side effects can be challenging for some patients even at low doses can be reduced by intake of lactase Renal dysfunction requires dose reduction. If it persists despite this, other renal causes should be considered, such as renal calculi
Deferiprone	Oral three times a day	3–4 hours	Needs to be taken in three divided doses for effectiveness due to its short half-life. This makes adherence challenging The relationship between dosing and iron balance is variable due to the dosing schedule and baseline liver iron concentration levels

Table 26.3 Iron chelation regimens with combination options.

Chelation option	Route	Decision-making process to choose best options
Desferrioxamine + deferiprone	Subcutaneous or intravenous + oral	• Preferred option for those presenting with myocardial iron with preserved ejection fraction, acute heart failure, or acute arrhythmias
Desferrioxamine + deferasirox	Subcutaneous or intravenous + oral	• Preferred option for those with severe liver iron with no excess cardiac iron
Deferiprone + deferasirox	Oral	• Preferred option for needle-phobic patients • Effective at cardiac iron removal • Helpful for patients with recurrent myocardial iron loading. For example, splenectomised transfusion-dependent anaemic patients

The lowest effective combination dose should be used.

Table 26.4 Optimal iron chelation according to age: current recommendations in the United Kingdom.

Patient age	Choice of chelation regime
Children under 2 years	• First choice: desferrioxamine 20–40 mg/kg 3–5 nights a week or • Deferasirox 7–21 mg/kg/day (unlicensed indication). Switch early if families are struggling with desferrioxamine to prevent worsening of iron loading
>2 years and <6 years	• First choice: desferrioxamine 20–40 mg/kg/day 5 days a week or • Deferasirox 14–28 mg/kg/day. Switch early if families are struggling with desferrioxamine
>6 years	• First choice: deferasirox 14–28 mg/kg/day or • Desferrioxamine 30–40 mg/kg/day for 5 days a week or • Deferiprone 75–100 mg/kg/day (unlicensed for sickle and transfused rare inherited anaemia)
Adults	• First choice: deferasirox – 14–28 mg/kg/day • Desferrioxamine 40–60 mg /kg/day or deferiprone 75–100 mg/kg/day

treatment during adolescence at university or work may differ from that when planning a pregnancy or raising a young family.

When to Start Iron Chelation Therapy

In regularly transfused patients, to avoid chelator toxicity, iron chelation is initiated when:

• Ferritin > 1000 ng/mL, or
• After 10–12 units of packed red blood cells, or
• >100 mL/kg/annum of packed RBC with HCT 0.6.

In nontransfusion-dependent patients, once ferritin has risen to 800 ug/L, patients should have an MRI iron assessment to confirm tissue iron overload. In nontransfused rare inherited anaemia, the ferritin threshold is set lower at 500 ug/L for MRI assessment. Chelation is initiated when liver iron concentration (LIC) is above >5 mg/g/dry wt.

Practical Tips for Clinicians

Desferrioxamine
• Avoid mean daily dose of >40 mg/kg in children.
• Avoid mean daily doses of >50 mg/kg in adult in routine use.
• Aim to reduce mean daily dose and try to avoid reducing the frequency of treatment when adjusting treatment.
• Always keep within the therapeutic index for desferrioxamine.

Therapeutic index is $\dfrac{\text{mean daily dose}\left(\text{mg/kg}\right)}{\text{Ferritin}} = <0.025$

Example: If a patient is on 40 mg/kg for 5 nights per week, with a ferritin of 3000

Mean daily dose $= \dfrac{40 \times 5 \text{ days}}{7 \text{ days}} = 28.5$

Therapeutic index: $\dfrac{28.5}{3000} = 0.009$

- Challenges to administration need to be addressed for good outcomes.

Deferasirox
- Start at a lower dose and build tolerance to overcome gastrointestinal side effects that include nausea, vomiting, stomach pains, and diarrhoea.
- Use lactase for those with lactose intolerance.
- Take with or after food.
- Consider *Helicobacter pylori* infection; reduce doses if there is abdominal pain and low serum ferritin.
- Reduce dose with a rapidly falling ferritin.
- Deranged liver function: often due to iron overload or intercurrent viral illness. No dose adjustment if <3 times upper limit of normal. Continue a lower dose if ALT <5 times upper limit of normal.

Deferiprone
- Start on a low dose and build tolerance to the desired dose.
- Maintenance dose is 50 mg/kg/day.
- If unable to tolerate a higher dose, then step back to the last tolerated dose.
- Neutropenia: be clear as to drugrelated or not.
- Discuss with the patient the risk of neutropenia/agranulocytosis versus the benefit when options are limited.
- In Diamond Blackfan anaemia, avoid as first line treatment due to the higher risk of agranulocytosis.

For good iron control, clinical teams need to know the rate of iron loading (ROIL) from blood transfusion to ensure the correct dose is prescribed to ensure an equal amount of iron excretion.

Calculation of ROIL Adults

$$\text{Rate of iron loading}\left(\text{mg / kg/day}\right) = \dfrac{\text{units of blood transfused} \times 200}{\text{weight} \times \text{days over which the blood was administered}}$$

Calculation of ROIL in Paediatric

$$\text{Rate of iron loading}\left(\text{mg / kg / day}\right) = \dfrac{\text{mL of blood transfused} \times 1.08}{\text{weight} \times \text{days over which the blood was administered}}$$

Practical Prescribing Tips

- Patients with average ROIL (0.3 mg–0.5 mg/kg/day) will require an average dose of chelation therapy.
- For desferrioxamine, this is 40 mg/kg 5 days a week and will maintain an iron-neutral state.
- Higher doses of desferrioxamine of 50–60 mg/kg 5 days a week will be required to achieve a negative iron balance.
- For deferasirox, a dose of 21 mg/kg/day is required for average ROIL.
- Those with rates <0.3 or >0.5 mg/kg/day will need dose adjustments. The necessary frequency of monitoring depends on the therapeutic regime used (Table 26.5).

Table 26.5 The necessary frequency of monitoring before and during iron chelation therapy depends on the regime used.

	Deferasirox	Deferiprone	Desferrioxamine
Prior to starting	Duplicate creatinine, ALT, urinalysis	FBC Creatinine, ALT	FBC Creatinine, ALT
Month 1	Weekly creatinine and urinalysis 2 weekly ALT	Weekly neutrophils	
Month 2 onward			
ALT	Monthly	Monthly	Monthly
Creatinine	Monthly	Monthly	Monthly
Urinalysis	Monthly		
Neutrophil		Weekly for 12 months then 2–4 weekly	
Audiometry	Annual (over 5 years)	6–12 monthly in combination chelation	Annual (over 5)
Ophthalmology review	Annual (over 5 years)	6–12 monthly in combination chelation	Annual (over 5)
Growth		Annual sitting/ standing height	3 monthly height/weight 6 monthly annual sitting/ standing height
Other		Zinc level	Zinc level Calculate therapeutic index Annual rate of iron loading

FBC, full blood count; and ALT, alanine aminotransferase
Source: Shah et al. (2021) / John Wiley & Sons.

Dose Adjustments for Comorbidities

Dose adjustments may be required in complex cases with comorbidities.

Renal Disease

Desferrioxamine
Reduced doses and frequency-can use up to three times a week and monitor for toxicity.

Deferasirox
Contraindicated if CrCl <60 mL/min: monitor closely and consider dose reduction with worsening renal function.
  Cr Cl < 30 mL/min: Avoid.

Established Dialysis
All three chelators can be used in low doses with close monitoring for toxicity.

Liver Disease

All three chelators can be used in Child Pugh A liver impairment and with raised transaminases.

Deferasirox
Contraindicated in patients with severe hepatic impairment (Child Pugh Class C)
  Caution in Child Pugh Class B.

Pregnancy

Low doses of desferrioxamine can be used from 20 weeks of pregnancy and during labour in patients with myocardial iron or liver iron loading to prevent decompensation.

If patients develop cardiac decompensation, then desferrioxamine should be started immediately regardless of the gestation of pregnancy as a lifesaving treatment.

Deferiprone and deferasirox are contraindicated. Transfusion-dependent patients should be started on desferrioxamine infusion at the onset of labour. This can be administered either subcutaneously or intravenously. The usual dose is 2 g over 24 hours.

Emerging Novel Therapies

There are a number of developments in the field of iron chelation, with new agents and targets.

SP-420 is a novel oral iron chelator of desferrithiocins class, which is undergoing early clinical trials in patients with transfusion-dependent beta thalassaemia. If it proves to be effective, it will certainly help improve adherence to medication given that it is longacting and needs less frequent administration.

Several early-phase clinical trials are seeking to correct iron homeostasis by targeting hepcidins, TMPRSS6, and ferroportin. Minihepcidins are hepcidin agonists, whilst treatments targeting inhibition of TMPRSS6 and ferroportin work by increasing plasma hepcidin levels and reducing iron absorption.

Bibliography

Cappellini, M.D., Farmakis, D., Porter, J., and Taher, A. (2021). *Guidelines for Transfusion Dependent Thalassemia*, 4e. Cyprus: Thalassemia International Federation.

Chauhan, W., Shoaib, S., Fatma, R. et al. (2022). Beta Thalassemia and the advent of new interventions beyond transfusion and iron chelation. *British Journal of Clinical Pharmacology* 88 (8): 3610–3626.

Makis, A., Voskaridou, E., Papassotiriou, I., and Hatzimichael, E. (2021). Novel therapeutic advances in β-Thalassemia. *Biology* 10 (6): 546.

Shah, F.T., Maharaj, R., and Pancham, S. (2023). *Standards for the Clinical Care for Children and Adult Living with Thalassemia in the UK*, 4e. London: UKTS.

Shah, F.T., Porter, J.B., Sadasivam, N. et al. (2022). Guidelines for the monitoring and management of iron overload in patients with haemoglobinopathies and rare anaemias. *Br J Haematol* 196 (2): 336–350.

Index

a

aconitase-1 (ACO1)   15
ACTH *see* adrenocorticotrophic hormone
       (ACTH)
activin receptor ligand   110
adrenal insufficiency   150
adrenocorticotrophic hormone
       (ACTH)   150
airway disease, chronic obstructive
       (COPD)   32
American College of Cardiology (ACC)
       guidelines   71
25 amino acid   17
   peptide hormone   11
aminocaproic acid   92
amiodarone therapy   150
anaemia   19, 49, 53
   anaemic patients   73
   congenital dyserythropoietic
       anaemia   166
   microcytic anaemia   49
   non-anaemic patients   73
   transfusion-dependent anaemia
       159, 161
anaphylactic or anaphylactoid
       reactions   41
angiodysplasia   62
angular cheilitis   47

b

anticoagulants   56, 72, 92, 99
antifibrinolytics   56, 92
   therapy   92
anti-inflammatory drug, non-steroidal   31
antiplatelet agents   31, 99
antiplatelet therapy   56
astrocytes   77, 78
atrial fibrillation (AF)   136
atrophic glossitis   47, 48
AUB *see* uterine bleeding, abnormal (AUB)
autoimmune gastritis   58

b

β-lactamases   18
biomarkers, non-invasive   148
bleeding
   duodenal Dieulafoy's lesion   61
   gastrointestinal   31
   intermenstrual   89
blood-brain barrier (BBB)   6, 78
blood loss
   lower gastrointestinal   58
   upper gastrointestinal   58
blood transfusion   55, 63
   allogeneic   98
   sporadic   119
B-lymphocyte-driven adaptive
       immunity   19

Iron in Clinical Practice, First Edition. Edited by Sue Pavord and Noemi Roy.
© 2025 John Wiley & Sons Ltd. Published 2025 by John Wiley & Sons Ltd.
Companion website: www.wiley.com/go/medicine5e

body mass index   144
bone disorder syndrome   66
bone marrow transplant   166
bone morphogenetic protein-6 (BMP6)   13
bone morphogenetic proteins (BMP)   14
British Society for Haematology (BSH)   53

c
calcium pyrophosphate deposition disease
    (CPPD)   155
Cameron lesions   58
cardiac comorbidities   150
cardiology, iron deficiency (ID) in
    diagnosis and uncertainty management,
        in individuals   73
    heart failure
        causes   71–72
        impact   72
        management   72–73
    iron replacement therapies   74
cardiomyocytes   11
cardiovascular compensatory
        mechanisms   95
catalase   6
cefiderecol   18
cell death   9, 120, 159
cell differentiation   6
cell proliferation   3, 6, 19
central nervous system (CNS)   77
Centre for Perioperative Care (CPOC)   53
cerebral venous sinus thromboses   79
chelation   161, 165
    parenteral desferrioxamine
        chelation   137
    therapy   148
chronic kidney disease (CKD)   32, 49
    non-dialysis-dependent
        (NDD-CKD)   65
CNS *see* central nervous system (CNS)
coeliac disease   58
colonic polyps, benign   31
colonoscopy   60
colorectal malignancy   49

combination chelation therapy
    clinical setting   168
    instructions, for clinicians   168–169
    iron chelation regimens
        with combination options   167
        with monotherapy options   167
        in United Kingdom   168
COPD *see* airway disease, chronic
        obstructive (COPD)
corticosteroids   31
cortisol, baseline   150
contraception, combined hormonal
        (CHC)   91
CPPD *see* calcium pyrophosphate
        deposition disease (CPPD)
C-reactive protein (CRP)   49, 54, 103
creatinine   54

d
deferasirox   137, 169, 171
deferiprone   137, 169
deoxyribonucleic acid (DNA) synthesis   3
desferrioxamine   168–169, 171
diabetes mellitus   147–148
Diamond Blackfan anaemia   165
diphtheria   20
divalent metal transporter-1 (DMT1)   13,
        14, 18, 78, 135
DNA synthesis   6, 19
drug metabolism   6

e
echocardiography   138
ejection fraction (EF)   71, 167
    left ventricular   138
    right ventricular (RVEF)   138
electrocardiogram (ECG)   138
electron transport   3
endocytotic vesicles (EV)   78
endogenous red cell   95
endothelial cells (EC)   78, 141
enterobacteriaceae   17
enterocytes, duodenal   11

enzyme activity, catalytic   3
epithelial cells   3, 14, 17
erythroblasts   130
  bone marrow   124
  development   129, 130
erythrocyte   6
erythroferrone (ERFE)   14, 131–132
erythropoiesis   14, 55, 129–130
  acquired abnormalities of   6
  IE
    ERFE   131–132
    erythropoiesis   129–130
    erythropoietin and iron   130–131
    ferrokinetic studies   131
  stimulating agents   108–109
erythropoiesis stimulating agent
  (ESA)   66, 108
erythropoietin (EPO)   14, 130–131
European Medicines Agency (EMA)   67
European Society for Medical Oncology
  (ESMO)   109
European Society of Cardiology (ESC)   71
extracorporeal blood circuit   66

f

faecal immunochemical testing
  (FIT)   50, 60
fatty liver disease, nonalcoholic   36
ferric carboxymaltose (FCM)   41, 65
ferric derisomaltose (FDI)   41, 65
ferritin   5, 13–16, 27, 31, 33–36, 38, 42, 49,
  54, 59, 63, 66, 67, 68, 71–73, 77, 78,
  80, 85, 86, 89, 92, 97, 101, 103, 108,
  109, 110, 117, 118, 119, 120, 126,
  130, 132, 135, 142, 143, 147, 149,
  160–161, 168, 169
ferrochelatase (FECH)   130
ferroportin (FPN/Fpn)   11, 13, 78
ferrous fumarate   39, 50
ferrous gluconate   39
ferrous sulphate   39
fibrinogenesis, accelerated   143
fibroids   90

fibrosis   159
FID *see* iron deficiency (ID),
  functional (FID)
follicle-stimulating hormone   148
fracture risk assessment tool (FRAX)   154
fragility fractures   153
FRAX *see* fracture risk assessment
  tool (FRAX)
free radicals   159

g

gastric antral vascular ectasia (GAVE)
  58, 60
gastric bypass surgery   58
gastritis   31, 72
gastroduodenoscopy, oesophageal (OGD)
  60
gastroenterology   65
gene regulation   6
genetic test, 'second-level'   127
global longitudinal strain measurements
  (GLS)   138
glomerular filtration rate, estimated
  (eGFR)   54, 68
glucose metabolism   147
glucose regulation, abnormal   147
glycated haemoglobin (HbA1c)   148
gonadotropin levels, non-elevated   148
growth hormone (GH)   150
gynaecology   65

h

haematology   86
haemochromatosis (HC)   12, 123,
  149, 153
  classification   125
  diagnosis   125–127
  frequency and penetrance   124–125
  genetic   161
  HFE-related   124–125
  pathogenesis   123–124
  treatment and prevention   127
haemodialysis session   66

haemoglobin (Hb)   53, 97
  content of reticulocytes (Ret HbC)   36
  glycated (HbA1c)   148
haemoglobinopathies   148
haemopoietic tissue   28
haemosiderosis   141
haemoxygenase-1 (HO-1)   13
haem-responsive gene-1 (HRG1)   13
haem synthesis   5
HCC *see* hepatocellular carcinoma (HCC)
heart failure (HF)   71
  chronic HF (CHF)   71
Helicobacter pylori
  gastritis   58
  infection   169
hepatic congestion   144
hepatic stellate cells (HSC)   142, 144
hepatocellular carcinoma (HCC)   141
hepatocytes   11, 142
hepcidin   11–18, 34, 40, 54, 59, 63, 67, 68,
     74, 83, 84, 86, 95, 98, 101, 103, 105,
     107, 124, 127, 131–132, 142, 143,
     153, 172
  antagonists   110
  block   104
  deficiency   123
  levels   37
H-ferritin   78
HFE test, first-level   127
H2-histamine receptor blocker   58
hiatus hernia   31
hip arthroplasty   155
HMB *see* menstrual bleeding, heavy
  (HMB)
hook osteophytes   155
hormone synthesis   6, 123
hyaluronan bound iron   13
hyperferritinaemia, metabolic   147
hypersensitivity reactions   41
hypogonadism   148, 150
hypoparathyroidism   10
hypophosphataemia   65, 66, 104

hypothyroidism   150
hypoxia-inducible factor-prolyl hydroxylase
     inhibitors (HIF-PHI)
  67, 110

i

ID *see* iron deficiency (ID)
idiopathic intracranial hypertension (IIH)   79
immune cells   11
immunity, nutritional
  and iron   17–18
  therapeutic interventions   18
inflammation
  arthritis   98
  bowel disease   58
  chronic   98
  disorder   16
  hepatic   144
insulin-like growth factor-1 levels
     (IGF-1 levels)   150
insulin sensitivity   149
intensive care units (ICU)   101
interleukin-6 (IL-6)   13, 17
intestinal cells   3
intrauterine device (IUD)   91
intravenous (IV) formulations   39
intravenous (IV) iron
  replacement therapy   40
  supplementation   56
  therapies   40–41, 73
IOL *see* iron overload (IOL)
iron
  accumulation   143, 160
  in body   3
    distribution   4
    essential functions   6
    ID   6
    IOL   6–9
    iron-containing proteins   4
  cellular   3, 14, 15
  status and susceptibility, to infections
    IOL and infection risk   20

iron deficiency and population
  health   19
on vaccine responses   20
iron-avid pathogen   20
iron-bound transferrin   3
iron-chelate complexes   165
iron chelation therapy   165
  administration of   166
  chelation regimens   166
  combination chelation therapy
      166–169
  dose adjustments, for
      comorbidities   171
  indications   165–166
  novel therapies   171–172
  prescription instruction   170
  ROIL
    adults, calculation   169
    in paediatric calculation   169
iron chelators   150
iron deficiency (ID)   6, 27
  in adults   35
  assessment of
    additional biomarkers   36
    ferritin thresholds   33–36
    hepcidin levels   37
    inflammation and liver disease   36
    red cell indices   36–37
  clinical situations
    COPD   32
    gastrointestinal bleeding   31
    heart failure   31
    renal disease   32
  functional (FID)   54
  in gastroenterology
    angiodysplasia   62
    assessment, in patients   59
    gastrointestinal causes   57–58
  in gynaecology
    and anaemia   92
    HMB   89–92
    impact   92–94

prevention   89
risks   94
impact
  non-pregnant premenopausal
    women   31
  paediatric population   30–31
  pregnancy, parturition and
    lactation   30
in intensive care
  clinical implications   103–104
  concomitant therapies, for anaemia
    104–105
  diagnosis   103
  intravenous iron   104
  iron homeostasis, in critical illness
    101–102
  patient blood management   104
investigations   59–62
management of, women with
    gynaecological bleeding
  blood transfusion   95
  oral iron supplementation   94
  parenteral iron supplementation   95
in neurology
  iron and neurocognitive
    development   79
  iron utilisation, in CNS   77–78
  management, with symptoms   80
  neurological symptoms   79–80
non-anaemic ID   27, 59
in obstetrics
  anaemia, in pregnancy   85–86
  diagnosis, in pregnancy   86
  fetal effects   85
  intravenous iron indications   86
  maternal effects   83–85
  postpartum anaemia   87
  risk factors   86
in oncology   111
  anaemia, causes of   107
  anti-anaemia agents   110
  blood transfusion   109

iron chelators (*cont'd*)
  cancer prevention 109
  diagnosis, in patients 108
  erythropoiesis stimulating agents
    108–109
  local policy implementation of
    109–110
  management of, anaemia 108
  in orthopaedics
    aetiology 98
    blood management, of patient 99
    diagnosis 97
    patient outcomes 98–99
    preoperative treatment 98
    without anaemia 100
  in preoperative patient
    causes, in surgical setting 54
    haemoglobin thresholds 53
    iron treatment 55–56
    management 55
    postoperative management 56
  in primary care
    causes of 48–49
    diagnosis 49–50
    dietary advice and prevention 51
    investigations 50
    overview 47–48
    treatment 50–51
  symptoms and signs 28, 30
  treatments
    administration of, oral iron 39–41
    adverse effects of, intravenous iron
      41–42
    individualised treatment 42
    intravenous iron therapy 40–41
    oral iron supplementation 39–40
iron deficiency anaemia (IDA) 33,
    65, 89
iron-deficiency-associated morbidity 27
iron-deficient erythropoiesis 27
iron demand, erythroid 16
iron depletion 27, 28, 39, 72
iron excretion 11, 169

iron homeostasis 9, 141
  systemic 11–12
iron-induced oxidative stress 148
iron overload (IOL)
  assessment of
    imaging 161–162
    ineffective erythropoiesis 160
    monitoring requirements, for at-risk
      patients 162
    repeated transfusions 160
    serum ferritin and iron
      studies 160–161
    transfusional 159–160
  on endocrine system
    adrenal function 150
    diabetes mellitus 147–148
    endocrine dysfunction
      assessment 151
    growth and bone health 150
    reproductive endocrinology 148–149
  and liver (heptatic)
    assessment 143–144
    histological patterns 141
    pathophysiology of, hepatic damage
      secondary 141–143
  and musculoskeletal system
    CPPD 155
    fracture risk 153–154
    joint pain 155
    management, in joints 155
    osteoarthritis 154–155
    osteoporosis 153–154
iron overload (IOL), in heart 135–136
  cardiac iron
    heart test 138
    MRI 137–138
  clinical presentation and management
    arrhythmia 137
    heart failure 136–137
    ventricular dysfunction 136–137
  iron and heart 135
  long-term management and prevention
    138–139

iron replacement therapies   39
iron response element (IRE) mRNA
        structures   15
iron salts absorption   39
iron sucrose (IS)   65
iron-sulphur clusters   5
iron-sulphur complex-containing
        enzymes   77
iron trafficking regulation   11
    cellular iron homeostasis   14–15
    hepcidin   11–12
    iron status assessment   15–16
    regulation of, hepcidin
        erythropoietic demand   14
        inflammation   14
        sensing iron concentrations   12–14
    systemic iron homeostasis   11–12
iron utilisation   5

j
joint aspiration   155

k
klotho   65
knee arthroplasty   155
koilonychia   47
Kupffer cells   36, 141, 142

l
liver biopsy   144
liver iron concentration (LIC)   143, 161, 168
liver sinusoidal endothelial cells
        (LSEC)   124
liver stiffness   144
L-type calcium channels (LTCC)   135
luteinising hormone   148
lymphocytosis, intraepithelial   59

m
macrophages   13
magnetic resonance imaging (MRI)
        137–138, 144
major adverse cardiovascular events
        (MACE)   67
malabsorption   58

malnutrition   58
maternal-to-fetal transfer   85
Meckel diverticula   58
Medicines and Healthcare products
        regulatory agency (MHRA)   42
menstrual bleeding, atypical   89
menstrual bleeding, heavy (HMB)   89
    causes of   89
    defined   89
    hysterectomy-specific complications   92
    investigation   90
    management
        anticoagulation modification   91–92
        haemostatic agents   92
        hormonal management   91
        hormonal preparations   91
    non-anaemic ID   92
    treatment   93
metabolic syndrome   36, 149
metacarpal hook osteophytes   155
metacarpophalangeal joints   154
metalloantibiotics   18
metalloproteins   5
metformin   149
microglia   77, 78
multi-drug resistant (MDR) pathogens   18
multiple contributory hormone
        pathways   150
myelodysplastic syndrome
        (MDS)   119, 166
myocardium   73

n
National Institute for Health and Care
        Excellence (NICE) guidelines   55
natural resistance-associated macrophage
        protein 1 (NRAMP1)   18
nervous system   8
neuroglia   77
neurons   77
neutrophil gelatinase-associated lipocalin
        (NGAL)   17
next-generation sequencing (NGS)   127

o

obligate co-receptor   65
oesophageal gastroduodenoscopy
      (OGD)   60
oesophagitis   31
oligodendrocytes   77
oral iron   55, 63
   supplementation   12, 39
osteoarthritis (OA)   153–155
osteopenia   150
osteoporosis   150, 153
   densitometric   153
   fracture   154
ovarian reactive oxygen species   149
oxygen transport   3

p

Parkinson's disease   79
patented R2 methods (FerriScan®)   144
pathology, gastrointestinal   98
patient blood management (PBM)   53
peptic acid disorders   31
peptide, cationic   17
percentage of hypochromic erythrocytes
      (%HYPO RBC)   36
peritoneal dialysis (PD)   65
pertussis   20
phosphorylation, oxidative   11
pica syndrome   58
pituitary dysfunction   148, 149
pituitary gonadotroph cells   148
pituitary hormone production   148
PIVOTAL   66, 67
plasmacytosis   59
platelet dysfunction   92
Plummer–Vinson syndrome   28
pneumococcal   20
point-of-care viscoelastic testing   56
polycystic ovarian syndrome
      (PCOS)   149
polyp, gastric   58
portal macrophages   141
primary care, iron deficiency (ID) in

causes
   older adults   49
   post-menopausal women
      and men   49
   pre-menopausal women   48
diagnosis
   haemoglobin   49
   iron studies   49–50
dietary advice and prevention   51
investigations   50
overview   47–48
treatment   50–51
pro-inflammatory cytokines   17
prolyl hydroxylase inhibitors   105
proteins, non-haem   6
proton pump inhibitor (PPI)   58
protoporphyrin IX (PPIX)   130
pyrophosphate crystals   155
pyruvate kinase deficiency   119

r

RAAS *see* renin-angiotensin-aldosterone
      system (RAAS)
randomised controlled trials (RCT)   66
rate of iron loading (ROIL)   160, 169
RCT *see* randomised controlled trials
      (RCT)
reactive oxygen species (ROS)   142
recombinant erythropoietin
      (rHuEPO)   104
rectal cancer   61
red blood cells (RBC)
   hypochromic   33
   indices   36–37
   maturation   7
   transfusion   104
redox reactions   11
red pulp macrophages   11
regulatory mechanisms   9
renal disease   32, 171
renal medicine
   intravenous iron isomaltoside *vs.* oral
      iron sulphate   69

iron use
  in haemodialysis patients 66–68
  in nephrology and safety
    considerations 65–66
  in non-dialysis-dependent chronic
    kidney disease 68
  in peritoneal dialysis 68–69
renin-angiotensin-aldosterone system
  (RAAS) 137
reproductive endocrinology 148–149
resection, duodenal 58
restless legs syndrome (RLS) 47, 79
restrictive transfusion policies 56
reticuloendothelial macrophages 3
reticuloendothelial system (RES) 33
RLS *see* restless legs syndrome (RLS)

s

Scheuer's grading 141
serious hazards of transfusion
  (SHOT) 55
seronegative inflammatory
  arthropathies 155
serum iron 161
SHOT *see* serious hazards of
  transfusion (SHOT)
sickle cell disease (SCD) 119
sideroblastic anaemia 165
signal intensity ratio (SIR) 144
soluble or serum transferrin receptor
  (sTfR) 36, 108
Staphylococcus aureus 17
staphyloferrins 17
surplus iron 5
symptomatic hypocalcaemia 150
syncytiotrophoblasts 11
synovitis, moderate 155
systemic anticancer therapy (SACT) 107

t

thalassaemia 12
  nontransfusion-dependent
    (NTDT) 161, 166

transfusion-dependent (TDT)
  118, 160
thyroid-stimulating hormone (TSH) 150
thyroxine levels 150
TIOL *see* transfusional iron overload
  (TIOL)
tissue accumulation 135
tissue Doppler imaging (TDI) 138
tissue transglutaminase (TTG)
  immunoglobulin A 50, 59
T or B lymphocytes 19
total dose infusions (TDI)
  single-visit 68
toxic nontransferrin-bound iron 159
tranexamic acid 56, 92
transferrin (Tf) 78
transferrin-bound iron 12, 161
  non-transferrin-bound iron (NTBI)
    13, 42, 132, 135, 142
transferrin iron 12
transferrin-mediated endocytosis
  (TFR1) 135
transferrin receptor (TFRC) 5, 13, 19
transferrin saturation (TSAT) 36, 54,
  108, 123
transfusion 87
transfusional iron overload (TIOL)
  causes 117
  consequences of 119–120
  distribution in, other diseases 119
  pathophysiology and effects 117–119
  prevention of 121
transient elastography (FibroScan®) 144
transmembrane serine protease
  matriptase-2 (TMPRSS6) 124
'Trojan horse' antimicrobials 18
trophoblastic tissue 86
tumour progression 108

u

ulcers
  duodenal 31
  gastric 31

ultrasound, transabdominal   90
ultrasound, transvaginal   90
uterine bleeding, abnormal (AUB)   89

V

venous thromboembolic disease   91
ventricular tachycardias (VT)   137
Vibrio vulnificus   20
video capsule endoscopy (VCE)   60
villous atrophy   59

vitamin D activation   153
vitamin D supplementation, activated   150
von Willebrand disease   91

W

World Health Organisation (WHO)
   6, 53

Z

Zrt-/Irt-like protein (ZIP)-8 or ZIP-14   13